Caregiver Survival 101:
Strategies to Manage Problematic Behaviors Presented in Individuals with Dementia

Lisa Byrd, PhD, FNP-BC, GNP-BC, Gerontologist

Caregiver Survival 101:

Strategies to Manage Problematic Behaviors Presented in Individuals with Dementia

Lisa Byrd, PhD, FNP-BC, GNP-BC, Gerontologist

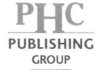

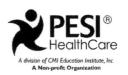

EAU CLAIRE, WISCONSIN
2011

PESI HEALTHCARE
PO BOX 900
EAU CLAIRE WI 54702-0900

Printed in the United States of America

ISBN: 978-0-9845254-4-7

PESI HealthCare strives to obtain knowledgeable authors and faculty for its publications and seminars. The clinical recommendations contained herein are the result of extensive author research and review. Obviously, any recommendations for patient care must be held up against individual circumstances at hand. To the best of our knowledge any recommendations included by the author or faculty reflect currently accepted practice. However, these recommendations cannot be considered universal and complete. The authors and publisher repudiate any responsibility for unfavorable effects that result from information, recommendations, undetected omissions or errors. Professionals using this publication should research other original sources of authority as well.

For information on this and other
PESI HealthCare products
please call 800-843-7763 or
visit our website at www.pesihealthcare.com

PUBLISHING
GROUP

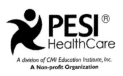
A division of CMI Education Institute, Inc.
A Non-profit Organization

Cover Photograph: Iain Sarjeant
Cover Design: Heidi Strosahl
Artwork: Josh Byrd

Preface

Yelling, throwing, hitting, incessant questioning, staying up all night (and all day too), crying, wandering, restless behaviors – having to contend with any of these behaviors on a daily basis makes it difficult for any caregiver to cope – especially if they are not able to reason with the person who is acting this way. It is impossible to rationalize with an irrational person – caregivers must learn to accept that fact. The key to diminishing the occurrence of, as well as calm, problematic behaviors in individuals with a diagnosis of dementia is to develop an understanding of the problem. And problems can be more tolerable if caregivers learn strategies to manage the behaviors and the person. Enhancing the quality of life for these individuals, while maintaining one's sanity, is the primary goal of care.

Disruptive behaviors are common among individuals who are suffering from dementia, and these behaviors can be distressing to anyone who must deal with these problems. Dementia is NOT a normal part of the aging process but is a problem which affects a significant number of elders. There are marked psychiatric and behavioral problems which occur in individuals who have a weak perception of reality and who experience memory loss as well as delusions or hallucinations. Everyday tasks and activities become progressively more difficult as a dementia affects an individual's ability to think, remember, and function independently. The day-to-day activities of communicating, driving, eating, bathing, dressing, and toileting become a challenge for individuals with cognitive impairment caused by any type of dementia, including Alzheimer's disease.

No two individuals with a diagnosis of dementia will exhibit the same behaviors nor will every individual respond the same to similar strategies for management. Every person with dementia will have their own unique presentation, but there are some common behaviors which have been observed in many individuals with dementia. Deciding what actions constitute a behavioral problem is highly subjective and the tolerability of behaviors – what actions caregivers can tolerate – depends partly on a person's living arrangements, with safety being the highest priority. Caregivers will decide what behaviors are acceptable and what behaviors require intervention. For example, an individual may wander off and become lost: wandering may be tolerable if a person lives in a safe environment – at home with locks or alarms on all doors and gates to prevent elopement or wandering off; however, if the person lives in a nursing home or hospital, wandering may be less tolerated because it disturbs other patients, puts an individual at risk for injury to self or from other patients, or interferes with the operation of the institution. Many behaviors such as wandering, repeatedly questioning, and being uncooperative are better tolerated during the day and are more difficult to manage in the afternoon and evening hours. These types of behaviors have been observed at this time of day, when individuals are less likely to be distracted and calmed. It is poorly understood whether this type of behavior, known as 'sundowning' (an exacerbation of disruptive behaviors at sundown or early evening), represents decreased tolerance by caregivers, or is a true exacerbation of behaviors and less response to redirection or other management techniques. In this book, there will be discussions about possible reasons why these behaviors occur and several suggestions for strategies to help caregivers manage problematic behaviors and calm upset individuals. But caregivers must remember that no technique will work every time and sometimes nothing will help. The information presented in the following pages is an attempt to provide caregivers, clinicians and families with the necessary knowledge to provide appropriate care for individuals with dementia, based on scientific research and common practice. The discussion will begin with an introduction to the problems and the common forms of dementia affecting behaviors, including their presentations. Also discussed will be ways to develop a plan of care, incorporating a holistic approach to management to include behavioral, environmental, and pharmacological strategies.

The author will present real life examples of geriatric behaviors and management strategies, both what has worked and what has not, based on over 25 years working in healthcare, over 13 years working as a Nurse Practitioner caring for elders in Nursing Homes, and from personal experience as a daughter caring for a mother who provided many examples of problematic behaviors. The strategies are based on research and best practices, as well as the author's professional and personal experiences. The strategies presented in this book are peppered with a belief that care for vulnerable individuals with dementia is an obligation for care to a person as an individual who is owed our respect and compassion.

Acknowledgements

'Caregiver Survival Guide 101' is a work meant to offer information, advice, and help for those who are in a place where I once was. I have 'been there, done that' and that is what I wish to share – my professional and personal experience. Writing this book helped me remember and grieve, as well as memorialize an outstanding mother.

I would like to express my gratitude to the many people who saw me through this book; to all those who provided support, talked things over, read, wrote, offered comments, proofreading, and design.

Above all I want to thank my husband, Ricky, my children – Josh and Sarah, my sister – Cathy Myers, and my niece – Brookleigh Allen, who were with me through Mom's life, illness, and death. They also lived through Mom's decline and played an active role in her care – we worked to provide support as well as encouragement to each other. It was a long and difficult journey for all.

I would like to thank PESI HealthCare for enabling me to publish this book – they had the belief that I could write a book worthy of helping others. I would also like to thank Steve Isaacson, Yvonne Kuter, and Heidi Strosahl for the arduous process of editing and molding this into a publishable work.

Thanks to Dr. Virginia Lee Cora, who offered her words of wisdom as well as provided support and encouragement during Mom's illness and in my efforts to write this book.

Last and not least: I beg forgiveness of anyone who has been with me over the course of the years and whose names I have failed to mention.

Table of Contents

This chapter presents a discussion of the various causes of dementia, including the physical as well as psychiatric changes and problems occurring. Current treatment plans to manage these disorders will be discussed including common diagnostic testing and management strategies (behavioral, environmental, and pharmacological).

We all know it happens; individuals with dementia are often still driving in the early stage of their disease. Families and other caregivers worry about safety – both of the individual as well as the community in which they drive. This chapter will provide some insight into how dementia, as well as normal aging changes, affect driving abilities in elders. There will be a discussion of how driving is often viewed as a form of self-reliance and independence and how cessation of driving impacts an individual's life. Strategies will be presented to assist caregivers in stopping individuals from driving when it is no longer appropriate or safe.

This chapter will include a brief discussion of 'Sundowning' and why it can occur in elders. Common problematic behaviors reported in individuals suffering from dementia will be presented including examples of triggers which may be causing the behavior to occur. Strategies to diminish the occurrence of behaviors as well as ways to manage behaviors will be reviewed, a brief discussion on why orientation theory is 'out-the-door', and the importance of validation and redirection – many examples of techniques will be reviewed including ways to decrease the bathing battle.

Caregivers of individuals with dementia often experience depression, anxiety, loneliness, isolation, and self-neglect. These issues can lead to stress and burn-out, even resulting in the caregiver dying before the one for whom they provide care. This chapter will present the signs and symptoms of caregiver stress and burnout as well as ways to manage and survival tips.

Alzheimer's disease and other dementias have a physiological cause, are progressive disorders, and are terminal diseases. Individuals who have these diseases often are not rational and many times are not allowed to choose the direction of their care – someone else makes the decisions for them because they often cannot think clearly and logically. There are many ethical issues to consider and this chapter discusses some of the issues surrounding truth telling and autonomy of cognitively impaired individuals. There will also be a brief discussion about justice – offering similar care to all no matter their financial status, race, religion, or cognitive ability.

Discussed in this chapter will be the legal issues which must be addressed in care of individuals with dementia, including assessing the decision-making ability of confused individuals, advanced directives, power-of-attorney – both medical and legal, guardianship, and important documents to locate. Also discussed will be the stages of dementia, common behaviors associated in the different stages, common triggers for behaviors, and strategies to managing the problems AND SURVIVAL TIPS.

In the final stages of a dementia (including Alzheimer's disease), there is a shift of care priorities and focus is on comfort care. Caregivers may experience grieving over the loss of the person even before their physical death. The complex and often disorderly progression of this terminal disease can make the journey to the person's final days difficult as the person reaches the stage where he/she requires complete care 24 hours a day, 7 days a week. Simple acts of daily care, such as bathing, feeding, turning, and cleaning the person; contrast with complex end-of-life decisions, such as whether to institute or continue life-prolonging medical care; and profound bereavement. Caregivers can learn to anticipate, remember, and reconnect with the person, which may ease the journey through care and grief.

A conclusion to our long journey will be shared and lessons learned from the experience.

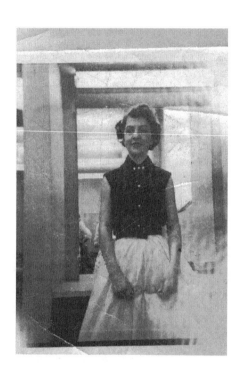

Chapter 1

Geriatric Behaviors in Individuals Suffering from Dementias – An Overview and Meet my Mom

In this chapter, there will be a brief introduction to the problems presented by individuals with a diagnosis of dementia, reasons why this problem will be epidemic as the elderly population explodes, and a discussion about reversible causes of confusion in elders which are not caused by dementia. The story of my Mom will begin here.

Introduction

Caring for a person whose perception of reality is altered due to a disease which causes dementia can be overwhelming. Each day brings different behaviors, new demands and may present opportunities as the caregiver copes with a person's changing levels of ability. Confusion and disorientation are common occurrences for individuals who have a diagnosis of dementia. This can make it increasingly difficult for the person to maintain a normal life due to the behavioral issues presented. Memory impairment and delusional beliefs are common in elders with dementia and may result in inappropriate behaviors in social situations or even at home resulting in difficult situations. Psychotic behaviors can also present in individuals with dementia which include hallucinations – usually visual, delusions, and delusional misidentifications.

Hallucinations are false sensory perceptions that are not merely distortions or misinterpretations

Delusions are beliefs that are untrue events but the events are not out of context with a person's social and cultural background

Delusional misidentification may result from a combined decline in visual function and recent memory problems: individuals may suspect that a family member is an impostor, believe that strangers are living in their home, or fail to recognize their own reflection in a mirror

Other troubling issues can include non-psychotic behaviors associated with dementia: agitation, wandering, sexual disinhibition, and aggression

Individuals who display physical or verbal aggression, which is associated with delusional misidentification, usually require a treatment plan which uses a combination of pharmacologic and non-pharmacologic treatments (Rayner et al, 2006). Abrupt changes in behavior may pose a greater challenge to management than cognitive decline for individuals with dementia and their caregivers. The nature and frequency of problematic behaviors varies over the course of an illness, but in most individuals, these symptoms occur more often in the later stages of disease (Rayner et al, 2006). Management of individuals with a diagnosis of dementia requires a comprehensive approach and incorporating a combination of strategies. It begins with an accurate assessment of symptoms, awareness of the environment in which symptoms occur, and identification of factors which precipitate symptoms as well as how the symptoms affect individuals and their caregivers. Non-pharmacologic interventions are the foundation of care and include creating a simplistic and safe environment, a predictable routine, counseling for caregivers about the unintentional nature of psychotic symptoms, and offering strategies to manage as well as cope with troubling behaviors. Approaches for an individual suffering from dementia involve a structured environment, behavior modification, appropriate use of sensory intervention, and maintenance of routines such as providing meals, exercise, and sleep on a schedule. Pharmacologic treatments should be governed by a "start low, go slow" philosophy: a mono-sequential approach to prescribing –

adding a single agent, titrating until the targeted behavior is reduced, side effects become intolerable, or the maximal dosage is achieved (Rayner et al, 2006). Goals of managing the care of individuals suffering from dementia and the behavioral issues which occur should include symptom reduction and preservation of quality of life.

Introduction to the Problem: Explosion of the Older Population

As of the year 2000, 16.3% of the entire US population was over 60 years of age, a 12% increase in this demographic group since 1990 (ASCLS, 2003). An increase in the geriatric population has been projected. In 2010 the elderly population had grown to 39 million, an increase of 17% since 2000. It is estimated there will be a rapid rise in numbers of elders between the years 2010-2030, increasing the elderly population to 69 million due to an aging baby boomer cohort. Elders are expected to increase by 75%. And between the years 2030-2050, the growth rate of elders is projected to increase another 14%, bringing the geriatric population to 79 million.

Aging & Characteristics of the Older Population

Aging is a process – it is universal, progressive, and unavoidable, occurring in all living individuals. Everyone will age as time marches on but all will age a bit differently. Aging is not a disease; it is the cumulative changes that occur in an individual over time. It is a series of biological, psychological, and spiritual changes (Cora, 2003).

The elderly population is currently healthier and living longer than generations before them. Most elders are able to live independently and manage their everyday activities but there are some conditions which can cause psychiatric problems in elders including dementia and depression. Normal aging does not cause a person to have problems with memory. A full medical work-up should be conducted on any older person who has problems with memory, has a personality change, or exhibits problematic behaviors in order to obtain an accurate diagnosis, to rule out treatable problems (which if appropriately treated may reverse the confusion) and develop an appropriate plan of care. The goal is to optimize an individual's quality of life and maintain, as well as encourage, as much independence as is possible.

The geriatric population is exploding in numbers and statistics report there are a number of medical issues which have not been as apparent as in previous years. Although the older population is much healthier than their parents, they are physically healthy but there is currently an increase in the number of individuals with some form of confusion. Confusion can be caused by dementia which often presents challenges in care. BUT not all older people will develop dementia. It is NOT a normal part of the aging process. Dementia is physical disease just like any other medical condition, such as hypertension and diabetes, but its symptoms are often exhibited as psychiatric or behavioral problems. (Byrd, 2003).

Of all the causes of dementia, Alzheimer's disease is the most common cause of dementia in the elderly population. As of 2010, only 10% of the population over the age of 65 had a diagnosis of Alzheimer's disease, meaning 90% did not. Healthcare providers, as well as society, must not assume an older person is destined to be confused or 'senile' as it was once termed, because this is stereotyping and this is not appropriate (and not true). Any older person who presents with confusion must be evaluated to determine if there is a cause of the confusion which can be treated and the problem reversed so the confusion will go away. Common reversible causes of confusion include depression, dehydration, infections, and medications, as well as other medical disorders.

Common (Reversible) Causes of Confusion in Elders

Anemia	B12 deficiency folate deficiency chronic kidney disease	not enough hemoglobin to carry oxygen to a person's brain
Cardiac Arrhythmias	Bradycardia	heart rate is too slow to circulate enough oxygen to a person's brain
Cardiac Arrhythmias	tachycardia atrial flutter atrial fibrillation	heart does not pump enough blood per heart-beat to get an appropriate amount of blood to a person's brain
Hypotension	blood pressure too low to get an adequate amount of blood to a person's brain	
Infections	a side effect of Urinary Tract Infections (UTI) or Upper Respiratory Infections (URI) in elders can include confusion	
Medications	confusion can be an adverse effect of medications such as benzodiazepines, barbiturates, pain medications, anticholinergic agents including diphenhydramine (benadryl), insomnia medications (sleeping pills – even ones you can obtain without a prescription: over-the-counter), steroids (prednisone, solumedrol), etc.	
Thyroid disease	Hypothyroidism and Hyperthyroidism	
Other	Brain tumor, Blood clots on the brain due to a fall, Meningitis, etc.	

Chapter 1 References

ASCLS (2003) Document: Role of the Clinical Laboratory in Response to an Expanding Geriatric Population. Position Paper. Retrieved May21, 2010 from http://www.ascls.org/position/ExpandingGeriatric.asp

Byrd, L. (2003). Terminal dementia in the elderly: awareness leads to more appropriate care. *Advance for Nurse Practitioners*. 11(9):65-72.

Rayner, A., O'Brien, J., & Schoenbachler, B. (2006). Behavior Disorders of Dementia: Recognition and Treatment. Journal of the American Family Physician. 73(4):647-652.

Meet Mom

My Mother was one of the most remarkable people I ever knew. She was an Emergency Room Nurse who worked the night shift. She was a single parent of two children and she was a very strong willed individual. She worked hard her entire life and was a very proud woman. She cared for almost everyone around her including her own mother until the day she passed away.

She was very independent, caring for her household, managing her own affairs, driving, and generally living her own life. We first realized there was a problem when her house was being foreclosed upon. Mom had always been a very savvy business woman but she had come to the conclusion that she was unable to pay all of her bills so she didn't pay any of them and decided to go to the casinos on the river instead. The problem became apparent when I discovered her house was in foreclosure. Now Mom had a retirement income, her car was paid off, and she should have been able to live on her income.

I lived on the other side of town where she lived, so I was always near but I had no clue there was a problem up until this point. When this realization came to light, we began to explore the problem. We managed to sell the house (at a bit of a loss – it was more run down than we realized) and moved Mom to a house 5 minutes away so I could help her with managing her financial affairs and help out if needed. She did well for a while but little things she said and did began to make us take notice and begin to worry. Children never want to think there is anything wrong with their parents and attribute a lot of the idiosyncrasy as normal part of aging – becoming a little more forgetful (all her friends were a bit forgetful too), getting lost going to the grocery store (after all she was in a different city), forgetting the main item she went to the store to get (heck, I do that), or staying up all

7

night (after all she did work night shift most of her adult life). We just put it off as getting older until the behaviors became more blatant.

The behaviors began to worsen and she became irritable when we asked her why she did-or didn't do-the things she did. She would change the subject, laugh it off, or start yelling and arguing when we asked her to explain certain things. Sometimes she could carry on as if nothing was wrong but other times she would do things that began to signal there was a problem – eating more junk food because it was easier but discovering she was unable to cook because she couldn't follow a recipe correctly; calling several times to ask me to bring her something from the store (not remembering she had already asked me to pick it up); and complaining about how rude and impatient the drivers were in the new town she lived – we will discuss the driving issues in a later chapter (this was really an issue). Nothing very indicative of the problem, just hints something just wasn't right.

Our story begins...

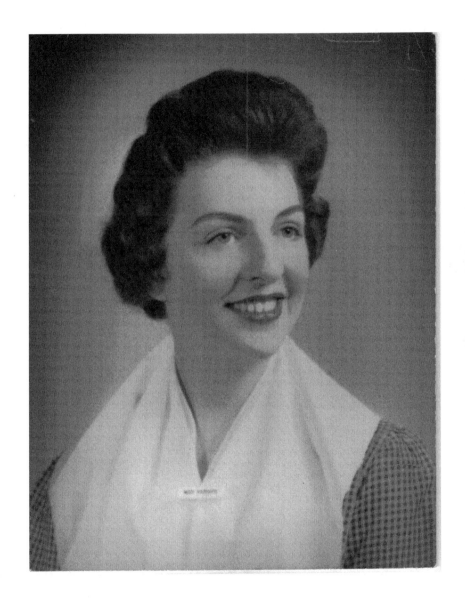

Chapter 2

Normal Aging, Depression, Dementia, & Delirium

This chapter covers a presentation of normal changes occurring in all older adults as well as diseases occurring in elders that affect memory and behavior. There will be a brief discussion of the pathophysiology, presentations, and ways to differentiate depression, dementia, and delirium in elders. This will assist in differentiating between the various causes of confusion in elders. Steps to appropriately diagnosing the problem will be discussed as the key to designing an appropriate plan of care.

Introduction

After the age of 20, people begin to lose brain cells a few at a time and a person's body starts to make less of the chemicals the brain cells need to work. As individuals age, thinking processes slow slightly and these chemical changes affect memory to some degree. Aging will affect one's memory by changing the way the brain stores information and making it harder for older adults to recall stored information. But short-term memories, as well as remote memories, are not usually affected by aging (FamilyDoctor, 2010).

After the age of 60, individuals experience some degree of neuron loss in their brains causing the size and weight of the brain to diminish slightly. (Alzheimer's disease Research, 2010) But this does not affect the ability of the brain to think, to reason, and to store new memories unless there is a pathological condition causing a problem. The quickness of thinking may slow as one ages, but the ability to think does not change. Most older individuals are able to think, function, live independently, and manage everyday activities throughout their lives.

It is not normal for an older person to be confused unless there is a cause. Some of the causes include illness and medications. There are some conditions which can cause mental health problems in aging individuals, for example dementia (including dementia of Alzheimer's disease) and depression. The main goal of care for elders experiencing problems in their ability to think and remember is to determine the cause of the confusion presenting in order to determine if there is a causative factor which can be addressed and the confusion be reversed. Any older person who has problems with memory should undergo a full medical work-up to rule out treatable causes, obtain an accurate diagnosis, and an appropriate plan of care created to meet each person's unique needs.

Causes of Memory Loss in Older Individuals

- Head Trauma
- Nutritional deficiencies (including anemia)
- Neurodegenerative diseases
- Thyroid disease
- Cardiac Arrhythmias (heart-rate abnormalities)
- Seizures
- Strokes or Transient Ischemic Attacks (TIAs)
- Electroconvulsive Therapy
- Infections/Illness
  - Urinary Tract Infections
  - Upper Respiratory Infections
- Dehydration
- Depression
- Medications
  - Benzodiazepines, Barbituates, etc.
- Alcohol Abuse
- Dementia (Alzheimer's disease & other dementias)

Normal Brain Pathophysiology

The quickness of thinking normally slows as an individual ages but a person's thinking processes are not generally affected. It may take longer to respond but the ability to respond is still intact in most elders. There is some degree of neuron loss in an aging brain, mainly in the brain and spinal cord, and most pronounced in cerebral cortex (Medline Plus, 2010). Neuronal dendrites atrophy with aging which causes an impairment of the synapses and changes in transmission by the chemical neurotransmitters. Growing older means there will be some atrophy within a person's brain and some changes within the workings of the brain but these changes generally do not affect the brain's functioning – including the ability to reason and remember. A simplistic view of memory storage is to compare memory storage to an electrical cord that transmits electricity – a switch is turned on, an electric charge runs down a cord, electricity is conducted the length of the cord, and electrical current reaches the object and activates the object to work; in a person – an individual sees an event, the event or memory is transmitted to the neuron – neurons are lined up end to end but not touching, the memory or impulse is conducted through the neuron, the end of the neuron (the dendrite) is activated to send a neurotransmitter (or chemical marker) to the next neuron which activates the next neuron to conduct the signal, and the action is repeated in sequence until the memory makes it to the brain's filing cabinet and stores the memory.

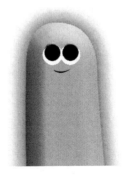

Memory Stored

Neurotransitter signals next neuron

- Next Neuron is activated
- Sequence is repeated until reaching the memory storage department where the Memory is stored

Signal travels through the Neuron

- Signal reaches the end of the Neuron (dendrite)
- Neural dendrite creates a chemical neurotransmitter (chemical marker)

Event occurs

- Memory is made
- Neuron is activated
- Signal created

Figure 1: Memory Storage

Most medical treatments are aimed at manipulating one or more of the chemicals in the brain to improve the brain's ability to think, reason, remember, and act appropriately. Mood is also one of the problem areas for elders who are suffering from confusion and can impact their quality of life as well as ability to think clearly. The main chemicals within the brain which play roles in mentation, ability to think, mood, and behavior include: dopamine, norepinepherine, serotonin, acetylcholine, glutamate, and possibly somatostatin and corticotrophin-releasing factors (Alzheimer's disease Research, 2010).

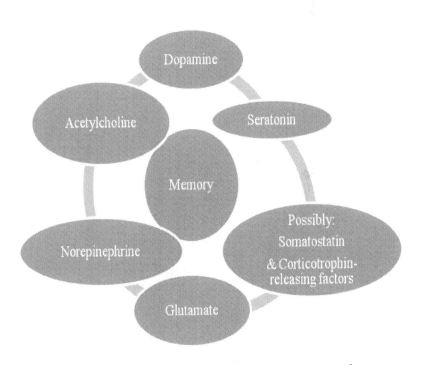

Figure 2: Chemicals within the Brain & Dementia

Discussed in the next chapter will be the ways in which medications are used to treat Alzheimer's disease and other dementias as well as medications used to improve quality of life. Developing an appropriate plan of care begins with an accurate evaluation of the problem and diagnosis while ruling out treatable problems.

Medical Work-up for Elders presenting with Confusion

Any elder who presents with confusion should undergo a full medical workup including physical examination, laboratory tests, and other diagnostic tests as determined by the healthcare provider. All of these tests are helpful in ruling out other problems, which are potentially reversible, and determining an accurate diagnosis. To assist in diagnosing the problem, practitioners should conduct an in-depth history of the elder's day-to-day functioning and any problems in behavior. It is important to obtain as much information from the person, first-hand. But it is also essential to obtain additional information from family and friends who may observe behaviors – this will provide a more reliable picture of the person and of issues.

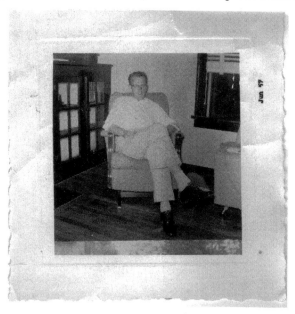

Laboratory test	Rationale or Potential Abnomality
• CBC	anemia or infection /reversible dementia
• Vit B 12	anemia/reversible dementia
• Homocystine	anemia/reversible dementia
• C reactive protein	inflammatory process
• Thyroid functioning	hypothyroidism
• Liver functioning	metabolic disorder
• Renal functioning	uremia/metabolic disorder
• Electrolytes/serum calcium	hypo/hypernatremia; hypo/hyperkalemia; hypo/hypercalcemia
• Glucose	hypoglycemia
• Lipid panel	vascular dementia risk factor
• Baseline EKG	cardiac anomalies /irregular heart-rate
• RPR	Syphilis

Diagnostic tests
- CT scan of the head
  - » Changes in later Alzheimer's disease (AD)
  - » Reduction in size of brain
- Magnetic Resonance Imaging (MRI)
  - » To rule out other causes such as Cerebrovascular Accident (CVA), Strokes, or tumors
  - » May see structural changes associated with Alzheimer's disease
- PET or SPECT scanning
  - » Difference in brain activity between normal brain & Alzheimer's disease (AD)
  - » Can help differentiate AD from other forms of dementia
- Other
  - » Neuropsychiatric testing (if appropriate)
  - » Central Spinal Fluid analysis (if meningitis is suspected)

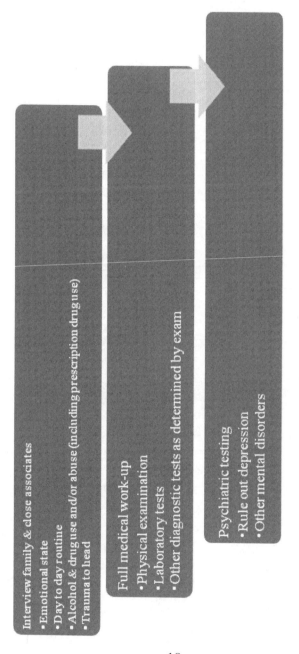

Interview family & close associates
• Emotional state
• Day to day routine
• Alcohol & drug use and/or abuse (including prescription drug use)
• Trauma to head

Full medical work-up
• Physical examination
• Laboratory tests
• Other diagnostic tests as determined by exam

Psychiatric testing
• Rule out depression
• Other mental disorders

Figure 3: Steps to Diagnosis

Depression

Depression can be confused with dementia in older individuals. Sometimes people over the age of 60 are treated as if they have a diagnosis of dementia when they become forgetful or present with **symptoms of self-neglect**: do not eat right, do not pay attention to personal hygiene, or have issues sleeping – too much or too little or exhibit behavioral problems. Elders can have many reasons to be depressed depending on their circumstances: many have chronic medical conditions and experience chronic pain or fatigue; many medications can cause an elder to feel bad; many have lost their loved ones and outlived their friends; and some have lost their homes due to inability to live independently and being placed in a nursing home setting. But being sad and sedentary is not an expectation of mood and level of functioning for people as they age. Depression is often under-diagnosed and under-treated in the older population.

Symptoms of Depression

Sad or Depressed Symptoms	Anxious Symptoms
• No interest or pleasure in things one used to enjoy, including sex • Feeling sad or numb • Crying easily or for no reason • Feeling slowed down • Feeling worthless or guilty • Change in appetite; unintended change in weight • Trouble recalling things, concentrating or making decisions • Problems sleeping, or wanting to sleep all of the time • Feeling tired all of the time • Thoughts about death or suicide	• Anxiety • Restlessness • Chronic complaints i.e., pain, constipation, insomnia, etc. • Muscle irritability • Irritability • Concentration problems • Headaches, backaches or digestive problems • Insomnia

Depression can lead to physical and psychological impairment as well as diminish quality of life. Older adults who are depressed and do not take care of themselves or of their medical conditions, will likely experience a decline in overall health. For example: an individual with a diagnosis of heart failure who does not adhere to a low salt diet, does not take his diuretic medication, and leads a sedentary lifestyle – the heart failure will worsen and the person will become sicker. Or if a diabetic person takes insulin and does not eat appropriately – the person's glucose level drops and possibly leads to a hypoglycemia episode. Self-neglect due to depression worsens an older person's overall health and diminishes quality of life. Depression can cause worsening of chronic medical conditions in elders, lead to increased healthcare costs, and increase the costs of healthcare for society since many of these elders end up in an acute care hospital where management is quite costly. Individuals who are not capable, or not willing, to care for their medical issues often end up in a long term care setting such as a Nursing Home where costs are expensive. Depression can also lead to suicide in elders who may succeed in a covert manner. For example, if an obese male with a history of congestive heart failures ingests a month's worth of cardiac medications over a short period of time or he was not taking any of his medications at all, he could become extremely ill and this could potentially lead to his death. Care must be taken to appropriately diagnose depression and treat the problem.

Delirium

Delirium is a sudden severe confusion with rapid changes in mentation – occurring over a few hours to a few days with markedly increased changes in level of consciousness including confusion and agitation. Delirium usually has a treatable cause, and once treated, the person returns to their baseline of level of consciousness, orientation, and functioning.

Common causes of delirium in elders

- Urinary tract infection (UTI)
- Upper respiratory infection (URI)
- Constipation
- Dehydration
- Hyperthyroidism or Hypothyroidism
- Depression
- Urinary Incontinence
- Urinary Retention
- Endocrine or other neurological problem
- Reduced Sensory input
    » Visual disturbances
    » Deafness
    » Sudden changes in environment
- Medications (over the counter as well as prescription)
    » Antidepressants with stimulating properties or caffeine can cause or exacerbate anxiety

Diagnosis of Exclusion: Once all other potential problems have been ruled out, an individual may be left with a Diagnosis of Dementia

Dementia is not a normal part of the aging process but does affect a significant portion of the elderly population. Some of the pathological causes of dementia include Alzheimer's disease, vascular disease, Lewy Body dementia, Parkinson's disease, and Pick's disease (Alzheimer's Association, 2006). Alzheimer's disease is the most common cause of dementia in elders and is a disease of the older population (Alzheimer's Association, 2010). Individuals who present with confusion or symptoms similar to Alzheimer's disease who are younger than 40 years, more likely have another diagnosis. Some of the familial forms of Alzheimer's disease can exhibit themselves in the 40s, but most individuals with Alzheimer's disease do not exhibit symptoms until they are in their 60s. The chances of acquiring Alzheimer's disease does increase with age: 1 in 12 people over the age of 65 and 1 in 3 over the age of 80 manifest the symptoms of the disease (AA, 2010).

The goals of treatment with any type of dementia (including Alzheimer's disease) are to slow the decline of cognition, maintain independence, and optimize an individual's quality of life. Environmental structuring, behavioral management, and medication usage are the main focus of care. They all must be addressed in order to provide quality care. Medications are often used but a pill is not the 'quick fix' to behavioral problems. Environment, routine, and behavioral management must be given attention in combination with any medication to appropriately care for elders with dementia. When a confused individual is placed in an environment which is over-stimulating with too much noise or too much activity or a person's routine is upset, the individual's world is upset and these factors can increase the likelihood the person will exhibit behavioral problems. Consistent environment and routine are very important to maintain equilibrium and decrease the incidence of behavioral problems in individuals with cognitive impairment or dementia.

Chapter 2 References

AARP. (2006). The pocket guide to staying healthy at 50+. Publication No. 04-1P001-A. Retrieved September 10, 2006 from www.ahrq.gov

Alzheimer's Association. (2010). About Alzheimer's disease. Retrieved February 10, 2010 from www.alz.org

Alzheimer's disease Research (2010). Retrieved February 21, 2010 from http://www.ahaf.org/alzheimers/about/understanding/brain-nerve-cells.html

Byrd, L. (2003). Terminal dementia in the elderly: awareness leads to more appropriate care. Advance for Nurse Practitioners. 11(9):65-72.

Cora, V. (2001) Elder Health. Community Health Nursing: Caring for the Public's Health. New York: Jones & Bartlett. p. 792-825.

FamilyDoctor.org (2010). Memory Loss With Aging: What's Normal, What's Not. Retrieved May 21, 2010 from http://familydoctor.org/online/famdocen/home/seniors/common-older/124.html

MayoClinic. (2006) Aging: What to expect as you get older. Retrieved October 14, 2006 from http://www.mayoclinic.com/health/aging/HA00040

Medline Plus. (2010). Aging changes in the nervous system. Retrieved February 21, 2010 from http://www.nlm.nih.gov/medlineplus/ency/article/004023.htm

Miller, K., Zylstra, R., Standridge, J. (2000). The geriatric patient: A systemic approach to maintaining health. American Family Physician. 61(4):1089-1106.

Reuben, D. B., Yoshikawa, T. T., Besdine, R. W. (2003). What Is A Geriatric Syndrome Anyway? Journal of the American Geriatrics Society. 51(4):574-576.

Senior Journal. (2006). Beers Criteria for mediations to avoid
    in the elderly. Retrieved October 14, 2006 from http://
    seniorjournal.com/NEWS/Eldercare/3-12-08Beers.htm
Tangalos, E. (2010). Diagnosing Alzheimer's disease: From a
    Mayo Clinic Expert. Retrieved February 19, 2010.

Chapter 3

Management of Alzheimer's disease

In this chapter will be a presentation on the stages of Alzheimer's disease: early, middle, late, and terminal stage, including the physical as well as psychiatric changes and problems occurring. Current treatment plans to manage this disorder will be discussed including common diagnostic testing and management strategies to include behavioral, environmental, and pharmacological interventions.

Introduction

Dementia has been around for a long time but it was not discussed as openly as it is now. In days gone by, families lived, worked, and died in the community where they were born. As grandparents grew older, when they were unable to care for themselves, either due to physical ailments or becoming 'senile', the family took them in and cared for them until their death. Many older individuals became confused and were told they had senility or organic brain syndrome. They were told this was a normal part of the aging process. But now this belief is no longer thought to be true; it is not normal to lose the ability to think. Only 10% of the population over the age of 65 have dementia, which means 90% do not. But dementia does impact society and the lives of the individuals with the disease as well as their families.

Previously, the impact of dementia in the older population has not been fully realized due to a common problem of stereotyping elders. This can be a form of **ageism** which views aging individuals with an expectation to become senile. This causes families to accept dementia as a normal part of the aging process and refrain from talking about this problem. Our current society is very mobile with people moving away for school or jobs, and not staying in the community in which they were born.

Society is now realizing the true impact of '**senility**' or dementia – the loss of mental functions such as thinking, memory, and reasoning which is severe enough to interfere with a person's ability to carry out the daily tasks of living. Dementia is not a disease itself, but rather a group of symptoms, caused by various diseases or conditions with symptoms which include changes in personality, mood, and behavior. It develops when the parts of the brain that are involved with learning, memory, decision-making, and language are affected by one or more of a variety of infections or diseases. The key to developing an appropriate plan of care is to differentiate the type of dementia, get an accurate diagnosis, and create an individualized plan of care. There are many causes of dementia in elders including Alzheimer's disease, Vascular disease, Lewy Body dementia, Pick's disease, Parkinson's disease, and other neurological disorders. The most common cause of dementia is Alzheimer's disease, accounting for greater than 50% of all dementias in elders (MedicineNet, 2010).

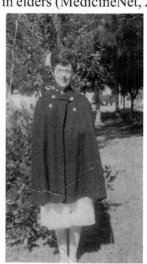

- Alzheimer's disease
- Vascular disease
- Lewy Body disease
- Pick's disease
- Parkinson's disease
- Other neurological diseases

Figure 4: Types of Dementia

Mom

Alzheimer's Disease

Alzheimer's disease was given its name in the early 1900's by Dr. Alois Alzheimer. Auguste D. was a woman who was brought to him for evaluation and treatment. She developed severe confusion, she was disorientated at home, hiding objects, and presented with symptoms of 'senility' or dementia – the loss of mental functions such as thinking, memory, and reasoning severe enough to interfere with her ability to carry out the daily tasks of living. She was very paranoid – accusing her husband of having affairs, which was not true since he took care of her 24 hours a day and never left her side. She was admitted to a German hospital and became a patient of Dr. Alzheimer. Upon examination, he found she was unable to remember her husband's name, the year, or how long she had been at the hospital. She could read but seemed to stress words in an unusual way and she did not seem to understand what she read. She sometimes became agitated and seemed to have hallucinations as well as irrational fears. She worsened over the span of a few years. Upon her death, Dr. Alzheimer examined her brain and found that it appeared shrunken and contained strange clumps of protein (plaques) and tangled fibers inside the nerve cells (neurofibrillary tangles) (MedicineNet, 2010). Auguste D was diagnosed with dementia and Dr. Alzheimer gave the disease its name. It is now clear that Alzheimer's disease (AD) is the major cause of dementia in elderly individuals.

The U. S. Congress Office of Technology Assessment estimates that as many as 6.8 million people in the United States have dementia, and at least 1.8 million of those are severely affected (MedicineNet, 2010). Research in the last 30 years has led to a greatly improved understanding of what this type of dementia is, risk factors for the disease, and how it affects the brain. Alzheimer's disease develops slowly and causes a gradual decline in cognitive abilities (Mayo Clinic, 2010). As the disease progresses, nearly all brain functions will be affected, including memory, movement, language, behavior, judgment and abstract reasoning. The rate of progression varies widely from person to person. In some individuals, severe dementia occurs rapidly, within five years after diagnosis. Often individuals are not diagnosed until they are in the middle stage of the disease and live for eight to 10 years longer. But some individuals can live up to 20 years after being diagnosed. People suffering from Alzheimer's disease will progress in the decline of their cognitive functioning as well as experience a decline in physical functioning. Most people with Alzheimer's don't die of the disease itself; they die of complications caused by the disease including pneumonias, urinary tract infections, or complications from a fall such as head trauma (Mayo Clinic, 2010). But Alzheimer's disease can cause death as the immune system shuts down and the body starts a cascade of multiple organ failure.

Financial Impact of Alzheimer's Disease

The number of Americans over the age of 65 is expected to grow. People are living longer than ever before due to advances in medical technology as well as social and environmental factors. This, in addition the exploding geriatric population created by the baby boomers aging and graying, will create a dramatic increase in the number of individuals with a diagnosis of AD. In 2000, an estimated 411,000 new cases of Alzheimer's disease were expected to develop and this number is estimated to have grown to 454,000 in 2010; future projections are an increase to 615,000 by the year 2030 and 959,000 – nearly 1 million – each year by 2050 (2009 Alzheimer's facts and figures).

Individuals suffering from Alzheimer's disease and other dementias are high users of healthcare and long-term care services incurring three times more costs than individuals without any form of dementia. The average annual costs for healthcare services are $33,007 for individuals with dementia, compared to $10,603 for individuals without dementia in the same age group (2009 Alzheimer's Disease Facts & Figures). There are additional factors which can contribute to the overall financial impact of dementia care on caregivers: average out-of-pocket expenses totaling $2,464 annually (co-pays for medications and office visits), plus supplies (mobility devices, incontinence supplies, and dietary supplements), and sitters or assistance for care. There are other factors to consider:

the impact of caregivers missing work, going in late, or leaving early to care for the individual with dementia (doctor visits, hospitalizations, or if the person is ill or having behavioral problems). Average out-of-pocket costs are highest ($16,689 annually) for individuals who are suffering from Alzheimer's disease and other dementias living in nursing homes and assisted living facilities. Alzheimer's and other dementias cost Medicare $91 billion each year and Medicaid spends $21 billion (2009 Alzheimer's Disease Facts & Figures). These figures will grow quickly as baby boomers begin to gray and this population explodes with many elders developing dementias. Since the greatest risk factor for developing AD is advancing age, many individuals with AD may have other age-related conditions, including hypertension, coronary heart disease, cerebrovascular diasease and diabetes, further increasing the cost of treating these individuals.

Pathophysiology of Alzheimer's Disease

The brain of a person with Alzheimer's disease often shows marked atrophy affecting every part of the cerebral cortex with the exception of the occipital pole which is often relatively spared. Microscopically, there are significant losses of neurons as well as shrinkage of large cortical neurons. There is loss of synapses in association with shrinkage of the dendritic arbor of large neurons. The hallmarks of AD are neuritic plaques and neurofibrillary tangles, but these can also be found in other neurodegenerative disorders as well and in individuals who do not exhibit symptoms of AD. Neurofibrillary tangles are found inside neurons and are composed of paired helical filaments of hyperphosphorylated micro-tubule-associated tau protein. The intracellular deposition may cause disruption of the normal architecture of the brain with subsequent neuronal cell death. Neuritic plaques and neurofibrillary tangles are not distributed evenly across the brain in persons suffering from AD, but are concentrated in vulnerable neural systems (Medscape, 2010).

29

Other pathological alterations commonly seen in the brains of AD individuals include neuropil threads, granulovacuolar degeneration, and amyloid angiopathy. Amyloid angiopathy is a distinct vascular lesion found in many AD brains. These deposits may cause the involved vessels to become compromised and hemorrhage causing further damage to the brain. Pathological criteria for a definitive diagnosis of AD found during an autopsy are a significant number of neuritic plaques and neurofibrillary tangles seen with microscopic examination. The most consistent neurochemical change associated with AD is a decline in cholinergic activity which is the main focus of treatment in AD. However, additional chemical imbalances have been found in AD including glutamate, norepinephrine, serotonin, somatostatin, and corticotrophin-releasing factors (Medscape, 2010).

Risk Factors for Alzheimer's Disease

Risk factors for Alzheimer's disease are variables associated with an increased risk for individuals of developing the disease – they are correlational and not necessarily causal. There are certain characteristics that increase the incidence of a person developing Alzheimer's disease which include lifestyle, environment, and genetic background. Some risk factors can be modified such as keeping diabetes in control; lowering cholesterol levels; and controlling blood pressure. Other risk factors cannot be modified such as a person's sex and genetic makeup. In general, most believe that Alzheimer's disease is caused by a combination of conditions and the effects of the various risk factors which overwhelm the natural self-repair mechanisms in the brain, thus reducing the brain's ability to maintain healthy nerve cells (Alzheimer's Society, 2010). Identification of risk factors for Alzheimer's disease is important because they can indicate lifestyle choices that can help reduce a person's chance of developing the symptoms of the disease.

Risk factors for developing Alzheimer's disease
• advanced age
• sex : women have a slightly increased risk of developing AD
• cognitive impairment
• poorly controlled hypertension
• poorly controlled diabetes
• elevated cholesterol levels
• low educational status
• certain genetic factors

(Lindsay, 2002; National Institute of Neurological Disorders & Strokes, 2010)

Age

Age is the most important risk factor, as the body loses the ability to repair itself and becomes less efficient. The loss of brain tissue varies from person to person and these differences contribute to the differences in an individual's susceptibility to develop and exhibit the symptoms of Alzheimer's disease. Aging individuals also have other risk factors for the disease which increase with age such as elevated cholesterol and being overweight. The older a person becomes, the higher the risk of developing the disease – 1 in 20 over age 65 develop Alzheimer's disease and 1 in 4 of those over age 85 are affected (Alzheimer's Society, 2010; NINDS, 2010).

Cardiovascular Disease

Cardiovascular diseases, including high blood pressure and high cholesterol levels, are also risk factors for both Alzheimer's disease as well as Vascular Dementia.

Diabetes

Diabetes Mellitus type II is a risk factor for Alzheimer's disease. It is believed that the utilization of glucose in the brains of individuals with Alzheimer's disease is impaired, somewhat resembling the situation in the bodies of people with Type II Diabetes Mellitus (Alzheimer's Society, 2010).

Mild Cognitive Impairment (MCI)

In certain individuals, there is a level of cognitive or memory impairment beyond that which usually occurs in individuals normally as they age but not truly a type of "dementia" or "Alzheimer's disease" – this is **mild cognitive impairment (MCI)**. It is estimated that up to 85% of people with MCI, often at a young age-in their early forties or fifties, will progress to develop Alzheimer's disease within ten years, making MCI an important risk factor for the disease. Researchers now know that the abnormal changes in the brain characteristic of Alzheimer's disease can begin to appear in people diagnosed with MCI more than twenty years before there are signs of dementia. Brain imaging may make it possible to detect the most at-risk individuals with MCI, and research is ongoing (Alzheimer's Society, 2010; NIA, 2010).

Low Levels of Formal Education

Several studies have shown that individuals with less than six years of formal education appear to be at increased risk of developing Alzheimer's disease. It is theorized that the brain stimulation associated with learning provides a protective effect for the brain and therefore more education provides greater protection. However, new studies challenge this, and it is now being suggested that there may be other factors associated with individuals who have a low educational background, such as an unhealthy lifestyle, which may account for the risk rather than low educational level itself (Alzheimer's Society, 2010; NIA, 2010).

Other Risk Factors

In addition to the risk factors previously described, the following are additional risk factors for developing Alzheimer's disease: Down's Syndrome, head injuries, inflammatory conditions (possibly reflecting immune system malfunction), and a history of depression, anxiety, and/or stress. Other risk factors that are also suggested include smoking, excessive alcohol consumption and drug abuse.

Down's Syndrome

Down's syndrome has also been linked to development of Alzheimer's disease (AD). The presence of extra material found in the genetic make-up of individuals suffering from Down's syndrome may lead to abnormalities in the immune system and a higher susceptibility to certain illnesses including AD. Individuals with Down's syndrome also experience premature aging and show physical changes related to aging about 20 to 30 years ahead of people of the same age in the general population. As a result, Alzheimer's disease is more common in people with Down's syndrome than in the regular population. Adults with Down's syndrome often are in their mid to late 40s or early 50s when Alzheimer's symptoms first begin (WebMD, 2010).

Head injury

Brain injuries at any age such as car accidents or falls, including those who have experienced repeated concussions such as individuals who have repeated seizures or boxers, football players or individuals who have undergone electroconvulsive therapy, are accepted by most clinicians as having an increased risk for developing Alzheimer's disease as they grow older.

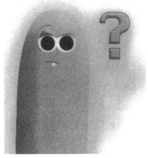

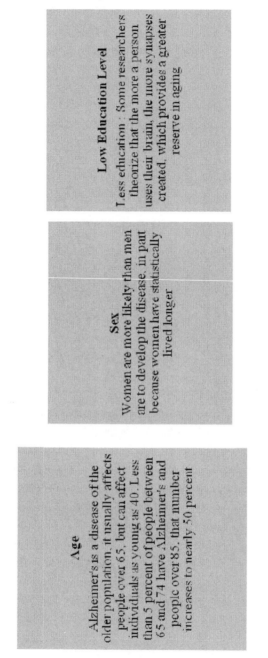

Figure 5: Risk Factors for Developing Alzheimer's Disease (part 1)

(Alzheimer's Society, 2010)

Other:
Down's Syndrome
Head Injury
Alcohol Abuse
Drug Abuse
Smoking
Depression
Inactive Lifestyle

Mild cognitive impairment
Individuals with mild cognitive impairment or have memory problems that are worse than what might be expected for people of their age

Genetic Factors
First degree relative with Alzheimer's disease-if familial type

Lifestyle
The same factors that put a person at risk of heart disease may also increase the likelihood that a person will develop Alzheimer's disease

Examples include:
• High blood pressure
• High cholesterol
• Poorly controlled diabetes

Figure 5: Risk Factors for Developing Alzheimer's Disease (part 2)

(Alzheimer's Society, 2010)

Genetic Factors

There are some individuals who carry a genetic factor which increases their likelihood of developing AD, but even having the genetic factor does not guarantee a person will develop the disease and exhibit the symptoms of the disease. Scientists have so far identified one Alzheimer risk gene called apolipoprotein E-e4 (APOE-e4) which is one of three common forms of the APOE gene; the others are APOE-e2 and APOE-e3. APOE provides the blueprint for one of the proteins that carries cholesterol in the bloodstream (Alzheimer's Association, 2010; NIA, 2010). Every person inherits a copy of some form of APOE from each parent and those who inherit one copy of APOE-e4 with the AD marker have an increased risk of developing Alzheimer's disease. Those who inherit two copies have an even higher risk. But inheriting two APOE-e4 genes with the AD marker does not mean an individual will develop the disease. Scientists do not yet know how APOE-e4 with the genetic marker for AD raises risk but believe that symptoms of the disease will be exhibited in these individuals who have this gene and the symptoms will appear at a younger age than usual-as early as in a person's in their 40s. Experts believe there may be as many as a dozen other Alzheimer risk genes (Alzheimer's Association, 2010). Routine genetic testing is not recommended due to the uncertainty of the findings and because true familial Alzheimer's account for less than 5% of cases.

Preventing Alzheimer's Disease: Build Cognitive Reserves & Exercise Your Memory

Building cognitive reserves is a lifelong process that begins in childhood when reading skills are learned. According to classic neurological theory, during early development, the human brain forms an enormous number of neurons, or nerve cells, but many of these cells will die as an individual ages. The neurons that survive do so by connecting with other neurons during the rapid-growth stages that occurs in childhood and adolescence. Learning more complex things and reading progressively more challenging books, creating art, playing games, and engaging in any mental activity will help form these vital neural connections that can last an individual's lifetime. These activities can also buffer individuals from cognitive decline later in life. Some believe that keeping the mind active throughout life may have a protective effect because the brain is like any muscle in the body – if you do not use it, you will lose it – and using the brain will preserve the functioning of the brain. Exercising the mind by learning new things and having fun with memory games are ways which are being recommended to prevent or even slow the cognitive decline associated with Alzheimer's disease. Researchers discovered that the more active individuals were, the less likely they were to develop Alzheimer's disease, for example engaging in activities such as playing a musical instrument, gardening, and playing mentally engaging board games (Alzheimer's Association, 2010). The benefit extended to those who were active between the ages of 40 and 60, so individuals are being encouraged to start building their intellectual muscle by learning new and different things as well as beginning stimulating hobbies which may benefit individuals regardless of the age the activity is started.

Preventing Alzheimer's disease through Memory techniques

- Learning new things
- Auditing classes at colleges
- Picture Memory
- Match the Cells
- Match the Words
- Sudoku Daily

Initiating Medications in the Early Stage of Alzheimer's is the Key to Slowing the Deterioration

Cholinesterase inhibitors in the early stage of Alzheimer's disease are the key to slowing the deterioration and preserving mental abilities. They are typically used to treat the early and middle stages of Alzheimer's disease because the decline in cognition is due to deterioration in the production of acetylcholine which accelerates over time, as more and more brain cells become damaged. Thus, the best chance to achieve a benefit for a person lies at the beginning of the disease even though the benefits of using cholinesterase inhibitors can be seen in all stages of the disease (Answers.com, 2010).

The benefits of cholinesterase inhibitors are judged by three patterns of the symptoms: a) in the early stage of Alzheimer's disease – improvement in a person's condition, possibly resulting in slightly improved cognition and memory (but not always); b) stabilization of the symptoms and slowing of the progression of the disease; and c) although it is inevitable the symptoms will worsen over time, slowing the disease advancement but at a rate that is slower than would occur if the drug(s) were not taken.

Stages of Alzheimer's Disease

There are common patterns of symptom progression that occur in many individuals with AD and there are many ways to stage the progression. Staging systems provide useful frames of reference for understanding how the disease may present in individuals. But it is important to note that not everyone will experience the same symptoms of the disease or progress at the same rate. People suffering from Alzheimer's disease die an average of four to six years after diagnosis but the duration of the disease can vary from three to 20 years (Alzheimer's Organization, 2010). The framework for this section is a system that outlines key symptoms characterizing four stages ranging from early to the terminal stage.

Early Stage of Alzheimer's Disease

The early signs of Alzheimer's disease (AD) are generally vague and not necessarily indicative of the disease. Occasionally forgetting words or names is common to most people, but this problem becomes more problematic and increases in frequency for individuals in the early stage of AD. Sometimes when an elder lives with a spouse or other relative, the symptoms may not be noticed as the problems because the symptoms gradually build over time and the relative accepts the changes as a normal part of aging or the caregiver compensates for the person. Elders with AD may begin having problems with language, for example they may use substitute words or use words that sound like the word they should have used as well as use words that mean something similar to the forgotten word. They sometimes change the subject, laugh off an incident, or even avoid talking to keep from making mistakes. They can become more subdued or withdrawn – especially in demanding situations. They may also put things in very odd places such as putting car keys in the freezer or placing a purse in the garbage can. They may ask questions repeatedly, make up stories, or hoard things. When frustrated or tired, they may become uncharacteristically irritable or angry. Their ability to think abstractly will begin to decline and they think more concretely. Examples of abstract thinking: they do not realize the reflection in the mirror is theirs and think someone is in their room; do not realize a message on the phone is not someone standing there talking to them so they search for the voice/person; or develop problems managing their financial affairs such as balancing a checkbook because these numbers are relatively abstract. The sequencing of numbers is another problem which develops, further causing difficulties managing finances, making change, and telling time.

Moderate Stage of Alzheimer's Disease

In the moderate stage of AD, organizational skills continue to decline and people lose the ability to think logically. They are unable to comprehend written material or follow written instructions. They often need help performing simple tasks such as grooming. Eventually, they will require help dressing because their confusion may cause them to put their shirt on backwards,

Early	Moderate
•Decreased attention span	•Increasing difficulty in sorting out names & faces of family and friends
•Less motivated to complete tasks	•Is able to distinguish familiar from unfamiliar
•Gets lost in familiar places	•Still knows own name
•Problems with language-use substitute words or words that rhyme	•No longer remembers addresses or phone numbers
•Misplace things or put things in strange places	•Can no longer think logically or clearly
•Trouble with abstract thinking	•Cannot organize own speaking or follow logic of others
•Changes in mood & personality-can become depressed or irritable	•Unable to follow written or oral instructions
•Apathetic, withdrawn, avoids people	•Unable to sequence steps, follow a series of instructions
•Anxious, irritable, agitated	•Arithmetic & money problems escalate
•Insensitive to others' feelings	•Disorientated
•Easily angered	•Season, day of week, time of day
•Frustrates easily, tires easily, feels rushed, surprises easily	•Poor short term memory
•Idiosyncratic behaviors start to develop	•Repeats questions repeatedly or tells the same story again and again
•Hoards, checks repeatedly, or searches for objects of little values	•Forgets recent events
•Forgets to eat or eats constantly	•Forgets names and words-may make up stories to fill in their own gaps in memory

Figure 6: Stages of Alzheimer's Disease (part 1)

Terminal

- Unable to swallow
- Increased incidence of choking/aspiration
- Becomes contracted in fetal position
- Increased incidence of pressure ulcers
- Incontinent of urine and feces
- Increased incidence of urinary tract infections
- Increased incidence of constipation/fecal impactions
- Decreased respiratory movements
- Increases incidence of respiratory infections & pneumonia
- Immune system fails
- Unable to fight off infection
- Recurrent Urinary Tract infections
- Recurrent Pneumonias
- Death

Late

- Mental abilities decline
- Personality changes
- Physical problems begin
- Complete deterioration of personality & movements
- Cognition
- Appears uncomfortable
- Can cry when touched or moved
- Can no longer smile
- Either unable to speak or speaks incoherently
- Cannot write or comprehend reading material
- Loses voluntary control of bodily functions
- Urinary and/or bowel incontinence
- Unable to walk, stand, sit up, or hold head without assistance
- Cannot swallow easily
- Pockets food or medicines in mouth
- Chokes easily
- Cannot move voluntarily

Figure 6: Stages of Alzheimer's Disease (part 2)

button it inappropriately, or even put shoes on the wrong feet. They may start having problems recognizing family members and friends or may mix up identities – thinking a son is a friend or a spouse is a stranger. Their short term memory is being lost and they do not recognize people as they age and change. They may not even recognize their own image in the mirror or recent pictures because, in their mind, they do not look like that old person; they still look like they did 10 to 20 years ago. They may become disorientated to time, day, month, season or even year as well as confused about where they are. Judgment is impaired and wandering behaviors become more common, making it difficult for individuals with moderate Alzheimer's disease to live independently (Mayo Clinic, 2010). Mood often becomes affected and they can exhibit more behavioral problems in the late afternoon and evening hours. They are 'forgetting they are forgetting', they begin to make up stories of occurrences and events which they convince themselves are reality, and they may become argumentative when attempts are made to orient them to reality or tell them they are incorrect.

Late Stage of Alzheimer's Disease

Transitioning from the moderate stage to the late stage, elders with Alzheimer's disease (AD) will lose the ability to smile or appropriately express their emotions, for example they may have a flat affect (a blank stare) or exhibit inappropriate emotions such as crying or laughing. These may occur as the mind is unable to interpret the individual's surroundings or the person loses the ability to appropriately make their bodies express the emotions they feel. They are unable to sit up without support and unable to carry out any of the activities of daily living without assistance: walking, sitting, eating, toileting, or even moving/turning over in bed. They usually become incontinent of urine and feces. They may no longer speak appropriately possibly reverting to one or two word responses, echo words said to them, saying mumbled or garbled words, making sounds such as grunts or moaning, nod to questions, or being unable to respond at all either looking in the caregivers direction or not looking at anyone at all. They are unable to recognize familiar faces including family members. Eating difficulties become worse with more problems in swallowing which can cause refusal to eat, choking, or aspiration. Sometimes elders with Alzheimer's disease forget the sequencing of the steps of eating and allow a bite of food to be placed in their mouth but they forget something is there and take a breat, leading to aspiration. They can even aspirate their own saliva and any aspiration has the potential to cause pneumonia.

Terminal Stage of Alzheimer's Disease

Alzheimer's disease (AD) is a disease which can cause death. In the final stage of the disease, the person loses the ability to understand, to respond to their environment, to speak and, eventually, the ability to control movement. Frequently they are unable to produce recognizable speech, although words or phrases may occasionally be uttered, moans, grunts, or occasional crying may be noted. They need to be fed and they are incontinent of urine and feces. They lose the ability to sit without support, the ability to smile or express emotions appropriately, and even the ability to hold their head up. Reflexes become abnormal, muscles grow rigid, and contractures can develop. Swallowing is one of the last abilities to become impaired and can lead to the person losing weight and potentially aspirating. The body's immune system begins to fail and the person is no longer able to fight off infections. The cumulative effect is the person will lose weight, develop contractures, have recurrent urinary tract infections (due to loss of ability to effectively empty bladder) and upper respiratory infections (due to decreased mobility, not taking deep breaths, and potentially aspirating oral secretions of food/fluids) as well as developing pressure ulcers (due to weight loss, urinary incontinence, and decreased mobility) which may become infected. The end result will be death due to a complication caused by Alzheimer's disease including pneumonia, sepsis, heart failure, renal failure, dehydration, or a combination of these problems

Diagnosing Alzheimer's Disease

In most cases, AD is a diagnosis of exclusion since there is no single test which can detect all forms of the disease. A full medical work-up is done and when no other diagnoses are found, and if the presentation is typical for Alzheimer's disease, then the diagnosis of Alzheimer's disease is made. It is generally diagnosed based on presentation of symptoms, findings on neurologic examination, and results from diagnostic tests (Mayo Clinic, 2010). There are certain forms of AD which can be detected through laboratory tests, the familial type and where blood markers are found, but there are many forms of AD that do not have blood markers. Certain individuals can be diagnosed based on Magnetic Resonance Imaging (MRI) tests and this is still controversial but researchers who are studying MRI as a diagnostic tool for Alzheimer's disease say the technique is promising, although there are no guidelines or recommendations yet for its use. In small studies, it has been reported that those in the early stage of Alzheimer's disease can be diagnosed with 84% accuracy based on measurement of the hippocampus (About.com, 2010). A diagnosis of Alzheimer's disease may be "probable," meaning that other causes of the symptoms have been ruled out and the most likely cause is Alzheimer's disease.

Initially, any individual who presents with confusion should have a complete physical exam-including laboratory tests, along with a detailed history of symptoms and medical history, medications, any recent injuries/falls, or surgeries. Examination by a neurology specialist may be done to assist in helping differentiate from other conditions such as Parkinson's disease, strokes, tumors and other medical conditions that may impair memory and thinking, as well as physical function.

Diagnosing Alzheimer's Disease

- Patient's medical and psychiatric history
- Information about the main problem, including any symptoms of confusion or difficulties in day to day functioning
- Information about other symptoms
- Past medical history
- Medications – both prescription and over-the-counter
- Psychosocial history – marital status, living conditions, employment, sexual history, important life events
- Mental state – any evidence of psychiatric illness, such as depression, anxiety, or memory impairment
- Family history (including any illnesses that seem to run in the family)

Neuropsychological Testing

Neuropsychological testing studies an individual's behavior and mood, and attempts to offer a definitive diagnosis when confusion presents in a person. It is utilized when an individual is having significant problems with memory, concentration, understanding, visual-spatial issues, and a variety of other symptoms. It is useful in differentiating between Alzheimer's disease and other various psychiatric problems, such as depression and anxiety, problems caused by medications, issues of substance abuse, strokes, and tumors. Neuropsychological testing is a lengthy process administered over an average of 8 hours which encompasses a comprehensive interview with the person. It may include tests to assess memory, language, the ability to plan and reason, and the ability to modify behavior, as well as assessments of personality and emotional stability (WebMD, 2010).

Mini-Mental State Exam

The Mini-Mental Status Examination (MMSE) developed by Dr. Marshal Folstein and Dr. Susan Folstein offers a quick and simple way to quantify cognitive function and screen for cognitive loss. It is not a diagnostic test but a test which can follow the progression of the disease in an individual when the test is administered periodically and that person's scores are compared – to show improvement in cognition, stabilization in cognition, or decline in cognition. It tests the individual's orientation, attention, calculation, recall, language and motor skills and each section involves a series of questions or commands. The individual receives one point for each correct answer. The administrator of the test is seated with an individual in a quiet, well-lit room. The individual is asked to listen carefully and to answer each question as accurately as he/she can. The test is not timed but the scoring is immediate. An individual can receive a maximum score of 30 points. In general, a score between 25 and 30 indicates adequate cognitive functioning: scores between 24 and 20 indicate mild cognitive impairment, between 19 and 10 usually indicate moderate cognitive impairment, and a score below 10 indicates severe cognitive impairment. The raw score may need to be corrected for educational level and age. Low scores may indicate the presence of dementia, although other mental disorders can also lead to abnormal findings. Physical problems can also interfere with interpretation if not properly noted; for example, an individual is unable to hear or read instructions properly, or may have a motor deficit that affects writing and drawing skills causing the scores to be abnormally low (Wikipedia, 2010). Despite the many free versions of the test that are available on the internet, the official version is copyrighted and must be ordered through Psychological Assessment Resources (PAR).

Clock Drawing Test

The Clock Drawing Test (CDT) is a simple test that can be used as a part of a neurological test or as a simple screening tool for Alzheimer's and other types of dementia. The test can provide information about general cognitive and adaptive functioning such as memory, processing information, and visual-spatial issues. It is highly correlated with the MMSE and a normal clock drawing almost always correlates with normal cognitive abilities (Kennard, 2006).

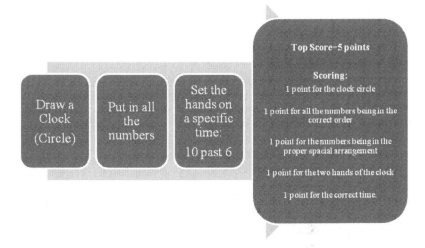

Figure 7: Clock Drawing Test

Mini-Cog Test

The Mini-Cog is a very simple and quick test which takes about 3 minutes to administer and is often used in situations to assist in identifying people who require further investigation into their clinical presentation. The test consists of a three item recall and a clock drawing test. First, a person is asked to remember 3 items and then is asked to draw a clock – the same as the Clock Drawing Test (CDT). Then the person is then asked to recall the three words. Scoring: If a person is unable to recall 3 words – he/she has some form of dementia; if able to name 1 to 2 words and able to perform an adequate CDT – the person probably does not have dementia; if able to name 1 to 2 words and unable to perform an adequate CDT – he/she is probably has some form of dementia; and if able to recall all 3 items – he/she probably does not have an Alzheimer's type of dementia or no form of dementia depending upon other symptoms presented by the person (Kennard, 2006).

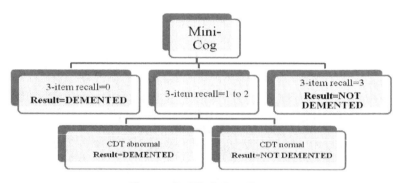

Figure 8: Mini-Cog Test

Treatment for Alzheimer's Disease

Treatment for Alzheimer's disease (AD) consists of slowing the progression of the disease, improving quality of life, and managing the problems caused by the disease. There are several different types of medications used to treat the associated memory loss, behavior changes, sleep problems, and the other symptoms of AD. A word of caution: all medications used in management of dementia, including AD, can have side effects, which can be even more pronounced in elders.

There are two classes of drugs that are approved by the Food and Drug Administration (FDA) specifically for treating Alzheimer's disease (AD). In the brain of individuals with AD, acetylcholine is destroyed too rapidly, making it difficult for the signals to be transmitted along the neural pathway. Cholinesterase inhibitors are used to slow this destruction and slow the progression of AD

48

as well as help improve cognitive symptoms. These medications work by preventing the breakdown of a chemical messenger in the brain called acetylcholine which is important for learning, memory, and attention. There are three cholinesterase inhibitors approved for the treatment of AD: Donepezil (Aricept) which is indicated and approved to treat mild, moderate, and severe Alzheimer's; Rivastigmine (Exelon) and Galantamine (Razadyne) which are indicated and approved to treat the mild to moderate stages of Alzheimer's disease. Rivastigmine (Exelon) is also approved to treat Parkinson's disease dementia. Side effects which have been associated with the use of the cholinesterase inhibitors include nausea, vomiting, diarrhea, weight loss, and dizziness.

The second class of drugs approved by the FDA to treat Alzheimer's disease is N-Methyl D–Aspartate Receptor Antagonists. There is only one medication in this class: Memantine (Namenda); it works by regulating the amount of another chemical messenger in the brain called glutamate which is made in excess in the moderate and late stages of Alzheimer's disease. Excessive glutamate causes interference with information retrieval and memory as well as behavioral problems. Namenda is indicated and approved by the FDA for treating the moderate to severe stages of AD and works by binding with the excessive glutamate. Side effects can include dizziness, confusion, headache, constipation, nausea, and agitation. Since Namenda works on a different chemical within the brain than a cholinesterase inhibitor, they are often used in combination.

Medications Indicated & Approved to Treat Alzheimer's Disease

Medication Class	Benefits	Medication/Dosing
Cholinesterase Inhibitors	*Slows the destruction of acetylcholine *May improve cognition: possibly improves the MMSE by 1-point *Cognitive benefits are sustained over 1 to 2 years (Average person untreated – dropped their MMSE score by 2 to 4 points annually)	Donazepril HCl (Aricept) *5 mg daily for 1 month then 10 mg daily **New 23mg dose available – it is also a once a day dose if appropriate in an individual who has been on 10mg daily for at least 3 months
		Ravistigmine (Exelon) *start @ 1.5 twice a day (abbreviated Bid), increase every 2 weeks 3mg Bid, then 4.5 mg Bid (max dose is12 mg daily); or Patch 4.6mg/24 hour applied daily for 2 weeks then 9.5 mg/24 hr applied daily
		Galantamine (Galantamin) *4mg Bid; increase every 4 weeks (max dose-12 mg Bid)
N-Methyl D – Aspartate Receptor Antagonists	*Regulates the production of glutamate and binds with excess glutamate *Calms agitation and other behavioral problems *May slightly improve memory retrieval	Memantine HCL (Namenda) *Start @ 5 mg daily for 1 week, increased to 5 mg twice daily for 1 week, then 5 mg in morning & 10 mg in evening for 1 week then to 10 mg twice a day **may stop @ 5 mg twice a day for individuals who have renal impairment

Other Medications

There are other medications commonly used in caring for individuals with a diagnosis of AD which are aimed at managing the behavioral and psychiatric symptoms including hallucinations, agitation, and sleep problems. However, none of these medications are indicated or approved by the FDA to treat dementia including AD. But all of these medications are commonly used and can be found in current literature discussing treatment of behavioral problems exhibited by individuals with dementia. The three main classes of medications include: a) Antidepressants which treat depression; b) Anxiolytics which treat anxiety and restlessness; and c) Antipsychotic medications which treat hallucinations, delusions, agitation, and aggression.

Antidepressants

Depression is common in individuals with a diagnosis of Alzheimer's disease or other types of dementia. Often antidepressant medications are used to treat this problem. The class of drugs most commonly prescribed in the elderly population is the Selective Seratonin Reuptake Inhibitor (SSRI) antidepressants because of their therapeutic efficacy and favorable side-effect profile (Salzman, Schneider, & Alexopoulos, 2010). They are highly selective in treating depression symptoms, are well known for their benign interaction and may offer individuals an equally effective, and far safer, alternative to conventional treatment with antipsychotic medications (Rosack, 2002). Antidepressants have been shown to be just as effective as an antipsychotic for calming agitation and treating psychotic symptoms in many older individuals with dementia (Pollock, 2007). There are other classes of antidepressant medications but the SSRIs are the class of choice in the geriatric population.

Anxiolytics

Anxiety is another common problem in individuals with a diagnosis of dementia. Anxiolytics are a class of anti-anxiety medications used to treat anxiety presented by individuals suffering from dementia. They work by calming and relaxing a person and may be prescribed in conjunction with other medications to relieve anxiety symptoms or slow the progression of dementia (eHow, 2010). Anxiolytics are good agents to use when a confused individual is unable to be consoled, redirected, or calmed and there is a potential for injury to self or others. They can produce side effects such as sleepiness, fainting, dizziness, blurred vision, confusion and potential falls due to the effects on an individual's balance. There are risks for use of this class if prescribed in high doses. There are potential interactions with alcohol or other drugs causing depression of brain functioning which can cause depression in respirations and potentially cause a person to stop breathing. Anxiolytics should be used cautiously but may be necessary when an individual is unable to function and has a poor quality of life due to anxiety, paranoia, or extreme delusions.

Antipsychotic Medications

Antipsychotic medications are not indicated for treatment of Alzheimer's disease but they are commonly used in individuals with a diagnosis of dementia to treat hallucinations, delusions, or extreme 'sundowning' behaviors. Antipsychotic medications are being used to decrease the psychosis or agitated behaviors associated with dementia to calm the racing thoughts, paranoia, and agitation. This allows a person to interact with other people, follow a routine, and be independent as possible. This class of medications must not be used as a chemical restraint which is use of a medication to quiet a person and make the person sedated. Antipsychotic medications may be used to enhance quality of life for an individual who exhibits distressing and agitated behaviors which endanger the person and/ or others. The benefits for using this type of medication must be weighed against the risks associated. It is important to note that there have been medical problems associated in older individuals who may take an antipsychotic medication. The adverse effects which can be caused by an antipsychotic medication may include an increased risk of strokes and death in individuals suffering from dementia, worsening of diabetes, worsening of cholesterol problems, increased risks for falls, and antipsychotics currently have a "black box" warning issued by the FDA about their use in older patients with dementia for increased risks of causing death. Antipsychotic medications can cause dystonia which are abnormal, repetitious, involuntary movements in individuals such as constant tongue protrusion, constant chewing, rocking motions, pill rolling, etc. If an individual develops dystonic movements, a medication's use must be re-evaluated to determine if it is in the person's best interest to continue use or if the medication should be discontinued. Appropriate laboratory monitoring is required with use of all of the antipsychotic medications including: laboratory tests to monitor liver and kidney functioning, Glucose and Hgb A1C to monitor status of diabetes, and cholesterol panels at least every 6 months.

Other Medications

There are additional medications used in the management of the symptoms of Alzheimer's disease and other dementias. Anticonvulsants have been used to manage behavioral problems presented in individuals with a diagnosis of dementia, although they have not been approved for this indication by the FDA. The most commonly used drug in this class is Divalproic Acid (Depakote), which has been used to treat epilepsy, bipolar disorder and migraine headaches. Psychiatrists observed that Depakote had certain side effects which included calming of anxious behaviors. It began to be used for these effects on mood and behavior in individuals with behavioral problems. This drug dampens the speed and frequency with which neurons fire. In addition to assisting in managing the symptoms of anxiety, agitation, and psychotic behaviors in individuals with dementia, scientists also think that Depakote may also inhibit the development of the plaques and tangle formation in the brains of Alzheimer's patients (Peterson, 2004). This medication should be used cautiously in individuals because it has the potential to cause sedation, falls, and orthostatic hypotension. There is a "black box" warning for liver damage which requires routine monitoring of liver function and drug levels. Be aware that a Depakote drug level in an individual's blood does not need to be in the drug's therapeutic range since it is not being used to treat seizures in these individuals – drug levels are being done to monitor for and prevent toxicity.

Other Medications commonly used to treat the problems associated with Alzheimer's disease

Many of the following medications are not indicated or approved by the Food and Drug Administration (FDA) to treat Alzheimer's disease or Dementia.

Medication	Geriatric Dosage Suggestions	Potential Side Effects of Medication
Antidepressants – Selective Seratonin Reuptake Inhibitors (SSRI) *indicated by the FDA to treat depression*		
bupropion (Wellbutrin)	75-100 mg once a day or twice a day	**Entire Class of SSRI: Weight gain, dizziness, somnolence, insomnia, decreased libido, tremors, akathesia, nervousness, sweating, and various gastrointestinal, as well as sexual, disturbances
duloxetine (Cymbalta)	20-60 mg once a day	
escitalopram (Lexapro)	5-20 mg once a day	
fluoxetine (Prozac)	10-20 mg once a day	
paroxetine (Paxil)	10-40 mg once a day	
paroxetine CR (Paxil CR)	12.5-37.5 mg once a day	
sertraline (Zoloft)	25-50 mg once a day	
venlafaxine XR (Effexor XR)	37.5-150 mg once a day	
Anxiolytics *indicated by the FDA for treatment of anxiety symptoms* – **Not recommended to routinely use anxiolytics**		
alprazolam (Xanax)	0.25-0.5 mg every 6 to 8 hours as needed	Sedation, falls, orthostatic hypotension & increased confusion
clonazepam (Klonipin)	0.125-2 mg every 12 hours as needed (*has a long half-life)	
clorazepapte (Tranxene)	3.75-15 mg every 8 hours as needed	

continued on page 56

Management of Alzheimer's Disease

Anxiolytics (***continued***) *indicated by the FDA for treatment of anxiety symptoms* – **Not recommended to routinely use anxiolytics**		
lorazepam (Ativan)	0.5-2mg every 6 to 8 hours as needed (*has the shortest half-life and is the drug of choice if absolutely necessary in elders with dementia)	

Antipsychotic medications *not indicated by the FDA for treating behavioral problems in elders with dementia; Indicated for use with agitation and psychosis in individuals with psychosis, bipolar disorder and other psychiatric conditions*		
aripiprazole (Abilify)	2-30 mg once or twice a day	Hypotension, seizures, hyperglycemia, worsening of diabetes, weight gain, headache, cataract formation, worsening of depression, & hyperprolactinemia
olanzapine (Zyprexa)	1.25-10 mg once a day at bedtime or twice a day	
quetiapine (Seroquel)	12.5-200 mg once, twice or three times a day	
risperidone (Risperdal)	0.25 to 1 mg once or twice a day	
ziprasidone (Geodon)	20-80 mg once or twice a day * QT prolongation, rash, hypertention * must monitor EKGs	*Antipsychotic medications have the potential to cause sedation, somnolence or insomnia, orthostatic hypotension, falls, strokes, diabetes, extrapyramidal symptoms, dystonic movements, myocardial infarction, and death **all patients receiving drugs in this class must have routine monitoring of liver & kidney functioning, Hgb A1C, Cholesterol
**all patients receiving antipsychotic drugs in this class must have routine monitoring of liver & kidney functioning, Hgb A1C, Cholesterol		

Seizure medication (used for its side effect of calming behavioral problems) *indicated by the FDA for treatment of seizure disorder and not indicated by the FDA for use of managing behavioral problems in elders with dementia		
divalproic acid (Depakote)	125-500 mg once or twice a day	Somnolence, dizziness, falls, orthostatic hypotension, increased confusion & liver toxicity *all patients receiving this medication must have routine monitoring of Liver functioning and Depakote levels

Other Alzheimer's Therapies

Several non-medication therapies are being used to help Alzheimer's patients cope with the symptoms of the disease.

Vitamin E. Vitamin E has been researched as a therapy for Alzheimer's disease because it is an antioxidant that is thought to protect nerve cells from damage. However, there is no proof it is efficacious and it is no longer recommended. It has also been noted that it can interact with other medications, particularly blood thinners.

Hormone replacement therapy (HRT). Some studies have suggested that postmenopausal women who are taking hormone replacement therapy have a lower risk of developing Alzheimer's disease. Estrogen, which is a female hormone, is thought to help nerve cells make connections, and interfere with the production of beta amyloid – a protein that is the main component in the plaques that lead to Alzheimer's disease. However, more recent research has found no improvement with HRT, and one study even suggested that estrogen use might actually increase the risk of developing

Alzheimer's rather than protect against it, as well as increase a person's risk for heart attacks, strokes, and developing breast cancer.

Sensory therapies. There is evidence that sensory therapies, such as music therapy and art therapy, can improve Alzheimer's patients' mood, behavior, and day-to-day function. By stimulating the senses, these therapies may help trigger memory recall and enable individuals with a diagnosis of Alzheimer's disease to reconnect with the world around them.

Alternative therapies. Some people have tried alternative remedies, including coenzyme Q10, coral calcium, huperzine A, and omega-3 fatty acids to prevent or treat Alzheimer's disease. However, there is no proven efficacy of these treatments to suggest recommending using any of these agents as an Alzheimer's therapy. And, because these are supplements, the FDA does not regulate them as it does prescription medications. Caution must be used since all dietary and nutritional supplements have the potential to cause dangerous side effects or interact with other medications individuals may be taking.

Lifestyle changes might help slow cognitive decline in people with Alzheimer's disease. For example, studies have shown that eating a Mediterranean diet (which is high in fish, nuts, and healthy oils) may reduce the risk of an individual developing Alzheimer's disease, and that exercise may improve the symptoms of the disease as well.

Researchers are looking into several new treatment options for Alzheimer's. One of the most promising Alzheimer's therapies in development focuses on beta amyloid. Researchers are trying to develop new therapies that prevent beta amyloid from forming, or break it down before it leads to Alzheimer's (Web MD, 2010).

Back to Mom's Story

Mom had some short-term memory issues off and on but the pattern of memory problems and behavioral issues were not truly consistent with Alzheimer's disease. So, we scheduled a Physical examination as well as had a CT scan done - there were some physical issues but no true evidence of Alzheimer's disease or a definitive diagnosis of Alzheimer's disease (she had a good day and had pretty good recent recall). Next we scheduled Neuro-Psychiatric testing. This was a long process; she didn't want to do it - she knew she was in a testing situation and knew some of her independence might be taken away if she didn't 'pass' the test. She was very nervous, and wasn't ready when I showed up to pick her up for the test, so I had to help her dress. We finally made it (not too late for the appointment though). They took her in for the testing (family members are not allowed in the room so as not to influence the results of the tests). After 3 hours (Neuropsychiatric testing lasts about 8 hours - must be performed in one day for consistency of results and by trained personnel) she emerged in tears, the testing had to be stopped because she was not able to continue; she was too upset. Now normally, the test is conducted in two parts: a morning session, a break for lunch and time for a short rest, and then an afternoon part. The results were not conclusive but we were given a diagnosis of 'Atypical Alzheimer's disease'.

Chapter 3 References

Alzheimer's disease facts and figures. (2009). Retrieved February 28, 2010 from http://www.alz.org/national/documents/summary_alzfactsfigures2009.pdf

About.com. (2010). MRI and Alzheimer's disease. Retrieved February 28, 2010 from http://alzheimers.about.com/lw/Health-Medicine/Conditions-and-diseases/MRIs-and-Alzheimers-Disease.htm

Alzheimer's Society. (2010). Alzheimer's disease: Risk factors. Retrieved February 28, 2010 from http://www.alzheimer.ca/english/disease/causes-riskfac.htm

eHow. (2010). Anxiety Medications Used in the Elderly with Dementia. Retrieved March 26, 2010 from http://www.ehow.com/facts_5761746_anxiety-medications-used-elderly-dementia.html

Kennard, C. (2006). Clock Drawing Test. Retrieved February 28, 2010 from http://alzheimers.about.com/od/diagnosisissues/a/clock_test.htm

Lindsay, J., Laurin, D., Verreault, R., Hébert, R., Helliwell, B., Hill, G., & McDowell, I. (2002). Risk factors for Alzheimer's disease: a prospective analysis from the Canadian Study of Health and Aging. American Journal of Epidemiology. 156(5):445-53.

Mayo Clinic. (2010) Alzheimer's stages: How the disease progresses. Retrieved February 27, 2010 from http://www.mayoclinic.com/health/alzheimers-stages/AZ00041

Mayo Clinic. (2010). Alzheimer's disease: Diagnosing. Retrieved February 28, 2010 from http://www.mayoclinic.org/alzheimers-disease/diagnosis.html

Mayo Clinic. (2010). Alzheimer's disease: Risk factors. Retrieved February 28, 2010 from http://www.mayoclinic.com/health/alzheimers-disease/DS00161/DSECTION=risk-factors

MedicineNet. (2010). Dementia. Retrieved February 28, 2010 from http://www.medicinenet.com/dementia/article.htm

Medscape. (2010). Alzheimer's disease: Pathology and Pathophysiology. Retrieved February 27, 2010 from http://www.medscape.com/viewarticle/553256_2

National Institute on Aging. (2010). Alzheimer's disease Fact Sheet. Retrieved May 21, 2010 from http://www.nia.nih.gov/Alzheimers/Publications/adfact.htm

Pollock, B. (2007). SSRI Comparable to Antipsychotic for Psychosis in Dementia. American Journal of Geriatric Psychiatry. Retrieved April 2, 2010 from http://www.medpagetoday.com/Geriatrics/Dementia/6632

Peterson, A. (2004). New Treatments For Alzheimer's Symptoms: To Curb Aggression, Paranoia In Dementia Patients, Doctors Turn to Schizophrenia Drugs. The Wall Street Journal. Retrieved March 26, 2010 from http://www.globalaging.org/health/us/2004/alz.htm

Rosack, J. (2002). SSRI Improves Behavior Symptoms In Demented Elderly Patients. Psychiatric News. 37(7). p 28.

Salzman, C., Schneider, L., & Alexopoulos, G. (2010). Pharmacological Treatment of Depression in Late Life. Retrieved March 28, 2010 from http://www.acnp.org/g4/GN401000141/CH.html

WebMD. (2010). Alzheimer's disease and other forms of Dementia. Retrieved February 27, 2010 from http://www.webmd.com/alzheimers/guide/alzheimers-dementia

WebMD. (2010). Down's syndrome and Alzheimer's disease. Retrieved February 28, 2010 from http://www.webmd.com/alzheimers/guide/alzheimers-down-syndrome

WebMD. (2010). Making the Diagnosis of Alzheimer's disease. Retrieved February 28, 2010 from http://www.webmd.com/alzheimers/guide/making-diagnosis?page=3

Wikipedia. (2010). MMSE. Retrieved February 28, 2010 from http://en.wikipedia.org/wiki/Mini-mental_state_examination#Interpretation

Chapter 4

Other Dementias: Lewy Body, Pick's Disease, Parkinson's Disease, and Other Neurodegenerative Disorders.

This chapter presents a discussion of the various causes of dementia, including the physical as well as psychiatric changes and problems occurring. Current treatment plans to manage these disorders will be discussed including common diagnostic testing and management strategies (behavioral, environmental, and pharmacological).

Introduction

Dementia is the loss of mental functions, including the ability to think, remember, and reason, which is severe enough to interfere with an individual's daily life. In addition to changes in memory, there can be changes in personality, mood, and behavior. Dementia is not a disease but a group of symptoms that is caused by various diseases or conditions. Although Alzheimer's disease is the most common cause of dementia, there are many other causes of dementia including vascular disease, Lewy Body disorder, Pick's disease, Parkinson's disease, and other neurological disorders. Some individuals will be suffering from a combination of dementias since certain dementias have similar risk factors, for example some individuals will have Alzheimer's disease (AD) in addition to another type of dementia.

Vascular Dementia

Vascular dementia is the second most common cause of dementia behind Alzheimer's disease, accounting for up to 20% of all dementias (MedicineNet, 2010). It is caused by brain damage due to cerebrovascular or cardiovascular disease and can be a result of a stroke or a hemorrhagic bleed within the brain. It often coexists with AD. The risks factors for vascular dementia increase with age and a sedentary lifestyle as well as other concurrent conditions including hypertension, hypercholesterolemia, diabetes, and obesity.

Risk Factors for Vascular Dementia

- **Increasing age** is one of the biggest risk factor for vascular disease and vascular dementia. Vascular dementia is rare before the age of 65. People in their 80s and 90s are much more likely to have this disorder than people in their 60s and 70s.
- **History of stroke** which causes brain damage appears to increase the risk of developing vascular dementia.
- **Atherosclerosis** is plaque build-up in the arteries and veins which narrows the blood vessels to the brain and impedes blood flow to the tissues. This increases the risks of strokes and brain damage and increases the risk of developing vascular dementia.
- **High blood pressure** or **Hypertension** puts extra pressure on blood vessels throughout the body including the brain. This increases the risk of vascular problems in the brain.
- **Diabetes** can leads to elevated glucose levels which can cause damage to blood vessels throughout the body, increasing the risk for strokes and other vascular problems in the brain.
- **Smoking** increases the risk of atherosclerosis and vascular diseases as well as vascular dementia.
- **High cholesterol**, which is elevated levels of cholesterol, increases the risk of developing vascular disease, especially in individuals who have high LDL (the bad cholesterol). These individuals are at an increased risk for vascular dementia, as well as having an increased risk of developing Alzheimer's disease.

(Mayo Clinic-Vascular Dementia, 2010)

Types of Vascular Dementia

Vascular dementia can have a gradual onset over a long period of time or can begin suddenly, frequently occurring after a sudden event such as a stroke. The symptoms may or may not worsen with time and the symptoms may improve with time. When the symptoms do worsen, they can progress in a stepwise manner, with the person showing gradual decline over time, or with sudden changes in a person's physical functioning or cognitive abilities. Unlike individuals with AD, people with vascular dementia often do not have personality changes except for depressive symptoms. Emotional responsiveness generally remains normal until the later stages of this type of dementia (MedicineNet, 2010).

There are several types of vascular dementia including multi-infarct dementia (MID), which is caused by numerous small strokes in the brain and Binswanger's disease, a rare form of dementia which is caused by a gradual diminishing of blood flow to the brain. MID typically affects multiple areas of the brain. The cause of damage to the brain in vascular dementia is impedement of the blood supply to brain tissue caused by an occlusion – a stroke – or caused by a hemorrhagic bleed within the brain. Essentially, the damage to the brain occurs due to either lack of blood flow or small clots blocking blood flow resulting in brain damage, called infarcts. Binswanger's disease is characterized by widespread damage to the brain with injury to multiple small blood vessels leading to increased atrophy within the brain. There can also be extensive lesions in the white matter or nerve fibers of the brain with this disorder. Binswanger's disease leads to brain lesions, loss of memory, disordered thinking, and behavior as well as mood changes. Individuals with Binswanger's disease often show signs of abnormal blood pressure, stroke, blood abnormalities, disease of the large blood vessels in the neck, and/or disease of the heart valves (MedicineNet, 2010). Other prominent features include urinary incontinence, difficulty with the ability to walk, clumsiness, slowness, lack of facial expression, and speech difficulty. Treatment of Binswanger's disease is symptomatic and may include the use of medications to manage hypertension, depression, heart arrhythmias, and hypotension (low blood pressure). There may be improvement of symptoms with episodes of partial recovery.

Symptoms of Vascular Dementia

The symptoms of vascular dementia can vary from one individual to another, depending on the portion of the brain that is affected. Adding to the confusion, Alzheimer's disease and vascular dementia frequently occur together. In fact, some believe that having both problems is more common than just having one disorder – Vascular dementia or Alzheimer's dementia (Mayo Clinic, 2010). Individuals with vascular dementia often experience:

- Confusion
- Agitation
- Memory impairment
- Unsteady gait
- Urinary frequency, urgency or incontinence
- Night wandering
- Depression
- Decline in organizational thinking
- Difficulty planning ahead
- Trouble communicating details sequentially
- Memory loss
- Poor attention
- Poor concentration

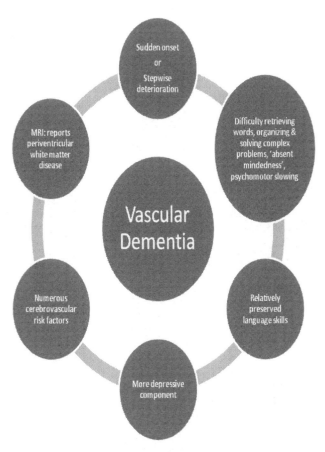

Figure 9: Vascular Dementia

Diagnosing Vascular Dementia

Diagnosing vascular dementia begins with a full medical work-up including a physical examination and laboratory tests. Radiological tests may be ordered to explore the possibility of strokes, cerebral hemorrhage, and brain tumors.

Diagnosing Vascular Dementia:

- Medical and psychiatric history
- Information about the main problem, including any symptoms of confusion or difficulties in day-to-day functioning
- Information about other symptoms
- Past medical history including hypertension, diabetes, hypercholesterolemia, and any brain injury including problems related to falls
- Medications – both prescription and over-the-counter
- Psychosocial history – marital status, living conditions, employment, sexual history, important life events
- Mental state – any evidence of psychiatric illness, depression, anxiety, or memory impairment
- Family history (including any illnesses that seem to run in the family)

Testing for Vascular Dementia

The following tests are often performed to rule out other conditions in individuals with memory impairment or individuals who are confused. One or more tests may be done in order to determine the cause of confusion. If a person is extremely confused, the individual may not be able to cooperate in order to have some of these tests conducted. A test's benefits must be weighed against the risks of conducting a test. For example if a person must be sedated to have the test done or if the person risks injury to self when having the test performed then a test may be more burdensome than beneficial and the test omitted. Sometimes it is beneficial to conduct psychiatric testing in addition to tests or in place of a test.

- **Computerized tomography (CT)** or CAT scan uses X-ray equipment to produce a cross-sectional image showing sections of a person's brain. Sometimes a contrast material may be injected to help highlight any abnormalities in the brain's blood vessels.
- **Magnetic resonance imaging (MRI)** uses radio waves and a strong magnetic field to produce detailed images of the brain. In some cases, contrast material may be injected to produce even more detailed pictures. Advances in MRI imaging and expertise in interpreting these results have proven to be an excellent tool for distinguishing between vascular dementia, Alzheimer's disease, and other dementias.
- **Positron emission tomography (PET)** is a scan of the brain after a person is injected with a low-level radioactive material which binds to chemicals that travel to the brain. This helps show which parts of the brain are not functioning properly. The test is painless and can be particularly useful in distinguishing between different types of dementia.
- **Doppler ultrasound** uses high-frequency sound waves to measure the direction and speed of blood cells as they travel through blood vessels – such as the carotid arteries which supply blood to a person's brain. A Doppler ultrasound of a person's carotid arteries can help detect blockages or narrowing vessels which impede blood flow to the brain.
- **Neuropsychological testing** assesses orientation, learning, recall, attention, calculation and language. Individuals with vascular dementia typically exhibit the same types of cognitive deficits as individuals with Alzheimer's disease. One major difference, however, is in memory function. Most individuals with vascular dementia do not experience short-term memory problems until later in the course of the disease unless there is a stroke in the exact area of the brain that controls memory.

(Mayo Clinic, 2010)

Treating Vascular Dementia

There is no cure for vascular dementia and there have been no drugs approved by the Food and Drug Administration (FDA) to treat this problem. Most medications that are used are designed to treat the symptoms of Alzheimer's disease, which often appears concurrently with vascular dementia. These medications have been shown to help reduce confusion as well as treat mood and behavioral problems in individuals with vascular dementia. The two classes of Alzheimer's medications used are:

- **Cholinesterase inhibitors** – donepazil (Aricept), galantamine (Razadyne) and rivastigmine (Exelon) – these are approved as treatment of Alzheimer's disease and work by slowing the destruction of acetylcholine, a chemical messenger which plays a key role in memory and judgment.
- **Memantine (Namenda)** has been shown to provide a modest benefit in individuals who have vascular dementia. Memantine works by regulating glutamate, a chemical messenger involved in information processing, storage and retrieval.
- **Antidepressants/Mood stabilizers** – Selective Seratonin Reuptake Inhibitors (SSRI) are antidepressants which may be just as effective as an antipsychotic medication for calming agitation and treating psychotic symptoms in older individuals with vascular dementia (Pollock, 2007).
- **Valproate** (Divalproic Acid or Depakote) is indicated to treat seizure disorders but also has an anti-aggressivity property which has demonstrated an ability to augment brain GABA and serotonin concentrations, thereby helping in the management of agitation/aggression in individuals with dementia (Guay & Lott, 2010).
- **Other Medications**: Efforts are also aimed at managing the risk factors for developing vascular dementia including managing hypertension, lowering cholesterol levels, controlling diabetes, and possibly thinning an individual's blood with use of aspirin or an anti-platelet aggregator medication, such as ticlopidine

(Ticlid) and clopidogrel (Plavix). This is to help prevent blood clots. Certain individuals may also be taking a blood thinner known as warfarin (Coumadin). None of these measures can reverse the problems caused by vascular dementia so most efforts are aimed at preventing further damage.

(Mayo Clinic, 2010)

Lewy Body Dementia

Lewy body dementia shares similar characteristics of both Alzheimer's disease (AD) and Parkinson's disease dementia (PDD). Like AD, it causes confusion. Like PDD, it can result in rigid muscles, slowed movement and tremors. Individuals with Lewy Body dementia (LBD) have microscopic protein deposits within the brain called 'Lewy Bodies' – abnormal structures in the mid-brain. These deposits, which have been found in nerve cells, can cause disruption to the brain's normal functioning, causing it to slowly deteriorate. They were first discovered in 1912 by Frederick Lewy, from which the name of the disorder was derived (HelpGuide, 2010)

The most striking symptoms of LBD are hallucinations, which can be one of the first signs of this disorder. Hallucinations may range from **visual hallucinations** which are seeing abstract shapes or colors to visions of animals and people or **auditory hallucinations** which are hearing sounds or voices which are not real. There can be instances where the individual with LBD has conversations with a visual hallucination – for example the person with LBD has a conversation with a deceased loved one. LBD is estimated to affect less than 1 percent of the population over the age of 65 (Crystal, 2009).

71

Risk Factors for Lewy Body Dementia (LBD)

LBD has several factors which appear to increase an individual's risk of developing the disease:

- Advanced Age – Most cases of LBD occur in individuals over the age of 60.
- Sex – LBD is more common in men.
- Heredity – family history; it appears to have a genetic link – if a person has a family member who has LBD, the risks for developing the disease are increased.

Diagnosing LBD

The criteria for a diagnosis of LBD is based on a person who has a progressive decline in the ability to think, as well as two of the following:

- Fluctuating alertness and cognition but generally good short-term memory
- Visual hallucinations
- Auditory hallucinations
- Parkinson's-like symptoms including tremors and pill-rolling motions, slow & rigid movements, and muscle stiffness
- Repeated falls due to the Parkinson-like gait
  - » Walking with short & shuffling steps, arms at sides and the person does not swing arms with walking, stooped posture with head looking down at feet, and shoulders hunched forward, which throws off a person's center of balance
- Sleep disturbances, including insomnia and the person acting out dreams
- Delusions or depression
- Fluctuations in autonomic processes, including blood pressure, body temperature, urinary difficulties, constipation, and difficulty swallowing
- Day-to-day symptom variability

Diagnosing LBD

- Medical history, including Parkinson's disease, and psychiatric history
- Information about the main problem, including any symptoms of confusion or difficulties in day-to-day functioning
- Information about other symptoms
- Medications – both prescription and over-the-counter
- Psychosocial history – marital status, living conditions, employment, sexual history, important life events
- Mental state – this is a series of questions that will be asked to determine if the person is experiencing any evidence of psychiatric illness, depression, anxiety, or memory impairment
- Family history (including any illnesses that seem to run in the family) especially Lewy Body dementia, Schizophrenia or Bipolar disorder

No single test can diagnose LBD; the diagnosis is made through the process of a medical work-up and eliminating or ruling out other diseases and conditions that may cause similar signs and symptoms. Tests may include:

Neurological exam – Should be part of the physical exam, assessing for signs of Parkinson's disease, strokes, tumors or other medical conditions that can impair brain function as well as physical function.

Mental status exam – Assesses an individual's memory and thinking abilities. Initially an abbreviated version should be done and, if warranted, a longer version with neuropsychological testing should administered by trained professionals. This can help distinguish normal from abnormal aging changes and may help identify patterns in cognitive functions that provide clues to the underlying condition.

Electroencephalogram (EEG) – If confusion comes and goes, an EEG may be recommended to help determine if the symptoms are caused by seizures or Creutzfeldt-Jakob disease, a very rare degenerative brain disorder more commonly known as mad-cow disease. This is a painless test which records the electrical activity in an individual's brain.

Brain scans – An MRI or CT scan can examine for evidence of stroke or bleeding, and is used to rule out the possibility of a tumor (see under Vascular Dementia – Diagnostic Tests).

(Mayo Clinic, 2010)

Treating LBD

Individuals with LBD are often difficult to manage due to the behavioral problems which the disease manifests. There is no cure for LBD; there are not even treatments which can slow the disease. Treatments are aimed at managing the symptoms, setting limits, and constructing a safe and structured environment.

Medications

- **Cholinesterase inhibitors** – Alzheimer's medications work by increasing the levels of acetylcholine, a neurotransmitter or chemical messenger in the brain believed to be important for memory, thought and judgment. They can help improve alertness, improve cognition, and may help reduce hallucinations and other behavioral problems.
  - The benefits are often small and sometimes not even noticeable
- **Parkinson's disease medications** can help reduce Parkinson's-like muscular symptoms in some individuals with LBD but can also cause increased confusion, hallucinations and delusions.
- **Other Medications** may help control behavior problems caused by a loss of judgment, increased impulsivity, and confusion. Possible medications include:
  - **Mood stabilizers** – Selective Seratonin Reuptake Inhibitors (SSRI) are antidepressants which may be just as effective as an antipsychotic for calming agitation and treating

74

psychotic symptoms in older individuals with dementia (Pollock, 2007).

- **Valproate** (Divalproic Acid or Depakote) – A medication indicated to treat seizure disorders that also has an anti-aggressivity property and an ability to augment an individual's brain GABA and serotonin concentrations. Valproate acid has been shown to be efficacious in the management of agitation/aggression in individuals with dementia (Guay & Lott, 2010).

- **Stimulants** (such as methylphenidate) are not commonly used but have been shown to be of some benefit in the management of explosive behavior in adults who have not outgrown their hyperactivity. They are also used to treat certain individuals who exhibit autistic-like behaviors with coexisting hyperactivity and aggression. However, in some individuals, these agents may actually worsen aggressiveness and self-injurious behavior (Guay & Lott, 2010).

- **Antipsychotic medications** are indicated to treat bipolar disorder and psychosis. They have been used to manage behavioral problems in certain individuals. They have been shown to help improve delusions and hallucinations BUT at least a third of the people who have LBD have a dangerous sensitivity to this class of medications. Reactions can be severe enough to be life-threatening or can be pronounced as seizure-like activity, severe psychosis, or worsening of confusion and agitation (haloperidol, risperdal, olanzapine, quentiapine). They should not be used to treat individuals with Lewy Body dementia.

- **Parkinson agents**: Levodopa is often used to treat the Parkinson-like motor symptoms but may increase the hallucinations and aggravate other symptoms such as agitation and delusions.

Managing Behaviors Associated with LBD: All Therapies must include Environmental Structuring

Since antipsychotic medications can worsen the symptoms of LBD, limit setting and a stable environment are paramount in keeping the individual with dementia safe:

- **Modify the environment.** Reducing clutter and distracting noise can make it easier for someone with LBD to focus and function.
- **Modify the response.** A caregiver's response to a behavior can make the behavior worse. To avoid increasing agitation, it is preferable not to correct or quiz a person with LBD unless the person's actions are dangerous to self or others. Reassuring the person and validating his or her concerns can defuse most situations.
- **Modify tasks.** Break tasks into easier steps and focus on success, not failure. Structure and routine also help people with LBD feel safe.

Parkinson Disease Dementia (PDD)

Parkinson's disease is a progressive disorder of the central nervous system which causes slowness of movements, compromise of balance, muscle rigidity, and tremors. The disease is caused by low levels of a chemical called dopamine, which activates cells in a person's brain that makes a person's muscles move. Individuals who develop Parkinson's disease earlier than 40 years of age usually do not develop dementia until late in life, usually after 70 years of age, while individuals who develop the physical symptoms of Parkinson's disease late in life, usually after the age of 60, tend to develop dementia relatively rapidly, usually within 5 years after onset of the disease. The key features associated with PDD are cognitive impairment including slowing in the ability to think, reduced attention span, and impairment of executive functions such as planning, organizing, and solving problems. An individual may become obsessional, experience loss of emotional control, and exhibit outbursts of anger. Certain medications may cause or aggravate delusions (false beliefs) as well as visual hallucinations. The person may experience language problems such as stuttering and slower speech but will not have difficulty finding the correct word (Mayo Clinic, 2010).

Risk Factors for Developing Parkinson's Disease

- **Age** – Middle-aged adults who develop Parkinson's disease very rarely experience the dementia associated with Parkinson's disease until very late in life (>70). Parkinson's disease ordinarily begins in middle or late life, and the risk of developing dementia associated with the disease increases if an individual develops Parkinson's disease after the age of 60. The progression is usually rapid over 2-10 years.
- **Heredity** – There appears to be a genetic link and having one or more close relatives with Parkinson's disease increases a person's chances of developing the disease, although an individual's risk is still less than 5 percent.
- **Gender** – Men are more likely than women to develop Parkinson's disease.
- **Exposure to toxins** – There has been an association with ongoing exposure to herbicides and pesticides which places a person at a slightly increased risk of developing Parkinson's disease dementia.

(Mayo Clinic, 2010)

Symptoms of Parkinson's Disease

Most of the symptoms of Parkinson's disease involve disruption of motor functions. Other symptoms include lack of energy, mood and memory changes, and pain.

Primary symptoms of Parkinson's disease

- **Bradykinesia** – slowness in voluntary movement such as standing up, walking, and sitting down due to a delay in transmission signals from the brain to the muscles which may lead to difficulty initiating walking. But this problem can also lead to more severe problems such as "freezing episodes" which is when a person is unable to move and stops once walking has been initiated
- **Tremors** often occur in the hands, fingers, forearms, foot, mouth, or chin; typically, the tremors take place when the limbs are at rest as opposed to when there is movement
- **Rigidity** or stiff muscle tone often produces muscle pain that is increased during movement.
- **Poor balance** – due to the loss of reflexes that help posture causing unsteady balance, which oftentimes leads to falls

Secondary symptoms of Parkinson's disease

• Constipation	• Loss of intellectual capacity
• Difficulty swallowing	• Anxiety, depression, isolation
• Choking, coughing, or drooling	• Scaling, dry skin on the face or scalp
• Excessive salivation	• Slow response to questions
• Excessive sweating	• Small cramped handwriting
• Loss of bowel and/or bladder control	• Soft, whispery voice

(HelpGuide, 2010)

Treatment of Parkinson's Disease

There is no cure for Parkinson's disease but there are several medications used to treat the symptoms of the disease:

- **Levodopa/Carbidopa (Sinemet)** – This is a combination of Levodopa (the chemical that patients with Parkinson's disease lack) and Carbidopa (a chemical that helps the levodopa reach the brain). Its effectiveness tends to decrease after several years and adjustments in dosing may be necessary.
- **Entacapone (Comtan)** is a medication which helps Sinemet work better when it starts to lose its effectiveness. It is also available together with levodopa and carbidopa in a combined product called Stalevo.
- **Dopamine agonists** [ropinorole (Requip) and pramipaxole (Mirapex)] enhance an individual's natural production of dopamine by stimulating the brain. These medications do not have as much risk of long-term side effects as levodopa and they have less chance of losing effectiveness over time in comparison to levodopa. However, there are potential side effects which include dizziness and hallucinations, especially in the elderly or in patients with dementia.
- **Monoamine oxidase inhibitors** [selegiline (Eldepryl and Zelapar) and rasagaline (Azilect)] increase the amount of dopamine available in the brains of individual's with Parkinson's disease. They can be very helpful in a small subset of patients with Parkinson's disease and often have fewer side effects than the dopamine agonists but can be harmful when used together with certain other medications, especially some types of antidepressants. Individuals can also develop critically elevated blood pressure when they take these medications and eat certain types of foods.

(HelpGuide, 2010)

Symptoms of PDD

Dementia is a less common feature of Parkinson's disease early in the disease process; only 20% of individuals who develop Parkinson's disease also develop Parkinson's disease Dementia (PDD). Parkinson's patients who experience hallucinations and more severe motor control problems are at risk for dementia. For those patients with Parkinson's disease who go on to develop dementia, there is usually at least a 10- to 15-year lag time between their Parkinson's disease diagnosis and the onset of dementia (HelpGuide, 2010). Recent studies have suggested that individuals who develop Parkinson's disease later in life will have a quicker onset of dementia – with over 50% of this population beginning to develop dementia within 5 years after the onset of the physical symptoms of Parkinson's disease.

Cognitive symptoms in PDD include the following:
- Slowed thinking
- Loss of decision-making ability
- Inflexibility in adapting to changes
- Disorientation in familiar surroundings
- Problems learning new material
- Difficulty concentrating
- Loss of short-term memory progressing to loss of long-term memory
- Difficulty putting a sequence of events in correct order
- Problems using complex language and comprehending others' complex language

Depression – Sadness, tearfulness, lethargy, withdrawal, loss of interest in activities once enjoyed, insomnia (not sleeping enough) or hypersomnia (sleeping too much), weight gain or loss

Anxiety – Excessive worry or fear that disrupts everyday activities or relationships; physical signs such as restlessness or extreme fatigue, muscle tension, sleeping problems

Psychosis – Inability to think realistically; symptoms can include hallucinations, delusions (false beliefs not shared by others), paranoia (suspicious and feeling controlled by others), and problems thinking clearly; if severe, behavior seriously disrupted; if milder, behavior bizarre, strange, or suspicious

Affect – Mask-like facial expressions

Speech – Slowing, generally hypophonic, some dysarthria and/or stuttering

Diagnosing PDD

- Medical and psychiatric history
- Information about the main problem, including any complaints of tremors, muscle rigidity, falls, or difficulty swallowing as well as any symptoms of confusion or difficulties in day-to-day functioning
- Information about other symptoms
- Past medical history including tremors or Parkinson's disease
- Medications – both prescription and over-the-counter
- Psychosocial history – marital status, living conditions, employment, sexual history, important life events
- Mental state – any evidence of psychiatric illness, depression, anxiety, or memory impairment
- Family history (including any illnesses that seem to run in the family) especially tremors or Parkinson's disease

---

Testing for PDD

There are no definitive tests which can confirm cognitive decline or dementia in Parkinson's disease. The most accurate way to measure cognitive decline is through conducting neuropsychological testing (eMedicine, 2010). Imaging studies which include brain scans such as Computerized Tomography (CT) scan and Magnetic Resonance Imaging (MRI) are of little use in diagnosing dementia in individuals with PDD. Positron-emission tomographic (PET) scan may help distinguish dementia from depression and similar conditions.

Treating Parkinson's Disease Dementia (PDD)

- **Anticholinesterase inhibitors**, specifically Ravistigmine (Exelon), are indicated to treat mild to moderate PDD. They are used to manage the cognitive decline such as the ability to think and remember; functional impairments such as activities of daily living including bathing, grooming and toileting;

and behavioral problems such as agitation and argumentative behaviors (Drugs.com, 2010).

- **Antidepressants** are aimed at treating mood disorders, as well as agitation associated with PDD and can include tricyclic agents, specifically the secondary amines (e.g., nortriptyline, desipramine), heterocyclic agents, or serotonin reuptake inhibitors (SSRIs), with the SSRIs being the most efficacious and safest in elders.

- **Anxiolytics**: Benzodiazepines may help treat severe anxiety, but side effects such as cognitive impairment and balance problems may be an adverse problem associated with their use. Behavior modification techniques are paramount to be used in conjunction with these medications in the treatment of anxiety. Buspirone is another alternative which is well tolerated but has not been studied in this population.

- **Antipsychotic** medications are not indicated to treat Parkinson's disease dementia, but have an indication to treat bipolar disorder. They have been used to manage behavioral problems in certain individuals. Clozapine is an older antipsychotic which has been used but is no longer commonly used due to the high incidence of associated adverse effects. Quetiapine (Seroquel) is the antipsychotic of choice in PDD because it has been shown to help with the cognitive decline as well as assist in management of psychotic symptoms (Medscape, 2001). Olanzapine and risperidone are also used but can worsen motor function and tremors.

- **Sleep disturbances**: Benzodiazepines can be helpful in the treatment of insomnia as well as rapid eye movement sleep behavior disorder. (Swanberg & Kalapatapu, 2010)

Pick's Disease/Frontotemporal Dementia

Pick's disease, or Frontotemporal dementia, refers to a group of dementias which result from hereditary disorders or can occur spontaneously e.g., occurring for unknown reasons. This disorder causes the frontal lobe of the brain and sometimes the temporal lobe of the brain to degenerate. In this type of dementia, an individual's personality, behavior, and language function are affected more than in Alzheimer's disease. And the person's short-term memory is less affected in Pick's disease (Merck, 2010). Diagnosis is based on symptoms and results of a neurologic examination, as well as the use of imaging tests to assess the brain damage. Typically, Pick's disease develops in individuals younger than 65. Men and women are affected equally and this disorder tends to have a heredity component – the incidence of occurrence of Pick's disease increases in individuals with one or more relatives with the disorder. These individuals have abnormal amounts or types of a protein called tau within their brains. In Pick's dementia, the frontal and temporal lobes shrink or atrophy and nerve cells are lost. These areas of the brain are generally associated with personality and behavior (Merck, 2010).

Risk Factors for Pick's Disease

The only risk factor for Pick's disease is family history; no other risk factors have been found.

Symptoms of Pick's Disease

Pick's disease (Frontotemporal dementia) is progressive, but how quickly an individual progresses to general dementia varies. Symptoms include inappropriate behavior, apathy, memory loss, carelessness, and poor personal hygiene. Death usually occurs within 2 to 10 years.

Symptoms of Pick's Disease or Frontotemporal Dementia

- Difficulty thinking abstractly
- Difficulty paying attention
- Poor recall

- Remains aware of time, date, and place
- Able to perform daily tasks
- Poor Personal Hygiene and Personal neglect

Changes in Personality and Behavior:
- Some people become uninhibited, resulting in increasingly inappropriate behavior:
  - speak rudely
  - abnormal increase in interest in sex
- Impulsivity and compulsiveness
- Repetitious actions
- Wandering or walking in the same location repeatedly
- May compulsively pick up objects or manipulate random objects
- May have an oral fixation and put objects in their mouth, may suck or smack their lips, or may overeat or eat only one type of food

Problems With Language:
- Difficulty finding words
- Difficulty using and/or understanding language (aphasia)
- **Dyarthria** – physically producing speech becomes more difficult
- Receptive aphasia – Some individuals cannot understand language, but speak fluently, although what the person says does not make any sense
- **Anomia** – Some have difficulty naming objects

- **Prosopagnosia** – Some have difficulty recognizing faces
- They often speak less and less or repeat what they or others say
  – Eventually, they stop speaking

Physical Changes
- In some people, muscles are affected and the individual may become weak and waste away (atrophy)
- Muscles of the head and neck are affected, making swallowing, chewing, and talking difficult

(Merck, 2010)

Diagnosing Pick's Disease (Frontotemporal Dementia)

- Medical and psychiatric history
- Information about the main problem
- Information about other symptoms
- Past medical history
- Medications – both prescription and over-the-counter
- Psychosocial history – marital status, living conditions, employment, sexual history, important life events
- Mental state – any evidence of compulsive behaviors, language difficulties, psychiatric illness, depression, or anxiety
- Family history (including any illnesses that seem to run in the family) especially Pick's disease or Bipolar disorder

The 5 Distinguishing Characteristics of Pick's Disease

- Onset before age 65
- Initial personality changes
- Loss of normal controls such as gluttony, hypersexuality
- Lack of inhibition
- Roaming behavior

(HelpGuide-Pick's disease, 2010)

Testing for Pick's Disease

The diagnosis of Pick's disease (Frontotemporal dementia) is based on symptoms, including how the symptoms develop. Observers may be helpful in diagnosing the disorder because the individuals who are suffering from Pick's disease may be unaware of their symptoms. A neurologic examination and neuropsychiatric testing may be conducted as well as radiological testing.

- Computed tomography (CT) and magnetic resonance imaging (MRI) are done to determine which parts of the brain and how much of the brain is affected. They can also be done to exclude other possible causes such as brain tumors, abscesses, or a stroke. However, CT or MRI may not detect the characteristic changes of frontotemporal dementia until late in the disorder
- Positron emission tomography (PET) may help differentiate Pick's disease from other dementias, but often PET is used only in research.

Treatment for Pick's Disease

There is no specific treatment for Pick's disease. Generally, treatment is focused upon managing symptoms and providing general support. Speech therapy may help those individuals with language problems.

- **Antidepressants/Mood stabilizers** – Selective Seratonin Reuptake Inhibitors (SSRI) are antidepressants which are used and may be just as effective as an antipsychotic medication for calming agitation and treating psychotic symptoms in older individuals with dementia (Pollock, 2007).
- **Valproate** (Divalproate Acid or Depakote) is indicated to treat seizure disorders but has been used in the management of agitation/aggression in individuals with dementia (Guay & Lott, 2010).
- **Stimulants** (such as methylphenidate) are not commonly used but have been shown to be of some benefit in the management

of impulsive behaviors in individuals who have not outgrown their hyperactivity. They are also used to treat individuals with autistic characteristics who have coexisting hyperactivity and aggression. However, in some individuals these agents may actually worsen aggressiveness and self-injurious behavior (Guay & Lott, 2010)

■ **Antipsychotic medications** are indicated to treat bipolar disorder and psychotic behaviors but may help improve delusions and hallucinations as well as calm agitated behaviors in individuals with Pick's disease (Pollock, 2007).

Other Dementias

Creutzfeldt-Jakob Disease: This rare disease, which causes a rapidly progressive dementia, can lead to a person's death within a year. The most common early symptoms for this disorder include memory loss and confusion. This disorder may resemble symptoms of other dementias. A variant form of Creutzfeldt-Jakob disease is thought to be acquired from eating beef contaminated with prions. This variant form of the disease causes a dementia similar to that of Creutzfeldt-Jakob disease, except the first symptoms tend to be psychiatric symptoms (such as anxiety or depression), rather than memory loss. There is no current treatment available.

HIV-Associated Dementia: In the late stages of human immunodeficiency virus (HIV) infection, the virus may directly infect the brain and cause damage to nerve cells resulting in dementia. Dementia may also result from other infections to which people with HIV infection are prone. Unlike almost all other forms of dementia, it tends to occur in younger individuals. This dementia may begin subtly but progresses steadily over a few months or years and usually occurs after other symptoms of HIV infection are evidenced. Symptoms include slowed thinking and expression, difficulty concentrating, and apathy, but abstract thinking and insight are generally not affected. Movements can be slow, muscles weak, and coordination impaired. When HIV infection is diagnosed or when mental function changes in people with HIV infection, computed tomography (CT) or magnetic resonance imaging (MRI) may be done to check for a brain infection or tumors. When confusion occurs in these individuals, a spinal tap, also referred to as lumbar puncture, may be performed to obtain a sample of cerebrospinal fluid for analysis and to check for infection, unless evidence suggests that pressure within the skull is increased. An individual's HIV infection may be treated with zidovudine and other drugs which sometimes produces dramatic improvement. However, because the infection is not cured, dementia symptoms may recur (Merck, 2010).

Dementia Pugilistica is a disorder which is also called chronic progressive traumatic encephalopathy and may develop in individuals who have repeated head injuries such as boxers, football players, etc. These individuals often develop symptoms similar to those of Parkinson's disease (e.g. tremors, muscle rigidity, etc), and some of them also develop normal-pressure hydrocephalus.

Figure 10 (pages 90-91) compares the symptoms of different types of dementia. Here is the 'note' regarding the Duration of Parkinson's dementia that accompanies Figure 10:

Note for Figure 10: Comparing the Different Dementias:

*In individuals with Parkinson's disease dementia, the onset is dependent upon the age of onset of Parkinson's disease: those who develop Parkinson's disease < 40 usually develop symptoms of dementia later in life; individuals who develop Parkinson's disease > 60 usually experience a more rapid onset of dementia symptoms.

(Hitti, 2006)

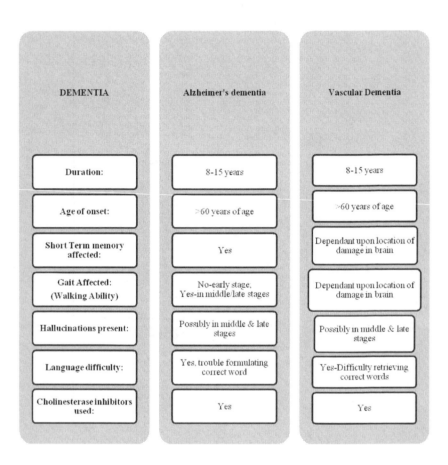

DEMENTIA	Alzheimer's dementia	Vascular Dementia
Duration:	8-15 years	8-15 years
Age of onset:	>60 years of age	>60 years of age
Short Term memory affected:	Yes	Dependant upon location of damage in brain
Gait Affected: (Walking Ability)	No-early stage, Yes-in middle/late stages	Dependant upon location of damage in brain
Hallucinations present:	Possibly in middle & late stages	Possibly in middle & late stages
Language difficulty:	Yes, trouble formulating correct word	Yes-Difficulty retrieving correct words
Cholinesterase inhibitors used:	Yes	Yes

Figure 10: Comparing the Different Dementias

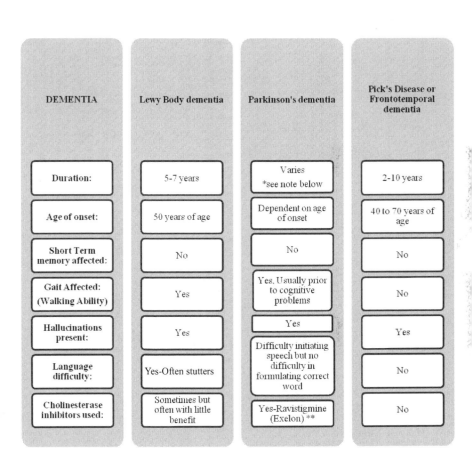

DEMENTIA	Lewy Body dementia	Parkinson's dementia	Pick's Disease or Frontotemporal dementia
Duration:	5-7 years	Varies *see note below	2-10 years
Age of onset:	50 years of age	Dependent on age of onset	40 to 70 years of age
Short Term memory affected:	No	No	No
Gait Affected: (Walking Ability)	Yes	Yes. Usually prior to cognitive problems	No
Hallucinations present:	Yes	Yes	Yes
Language difficulty:	Yes-Often stutters	Difficulty initiating speech but no difficulty in formulating correct word	No
Cholinesterase inhibitors used:	Sometimes but often with little benefit	Yes-Ravistigmine (Exelon) **	No

Figure 10: Comparing the Different Dementias

Chapter 4 References

eMedicine. (2010). Parkinson's disease dementia. Retrieved
April 2, 2010 from http://www.emedicinehealth.com/
parkinson_disease_dementia/page3_em.htm

Crystal, H. (2009). Dementia with Lewy Bodies. eMedicine
Retrieved May 21, 2010 from http://emedicine.medscape.
com/article/1135041-overview

Drugs.com (2010). FDA Approves the First Treatment for
Dementia of Parkinson's Disease. Retrieved April 2, 2010
from http://www.drugs.com/news/fda-approves-first-
dementia-parkinson-s-1842.html

HelpGuide. (2010). Lewy Body dementia. Retrieved March 31,
2010 from http://www.helpguide.org/elder/lewy_body_
disease.htm

HelpGuide. (2010). Parkinson's disease dementia. Retrieved
April 2, 2010 from http://www.helpguide.org/elder/
parkinsons_disease.htm

HelpGuide. (2010). Pick's disease. Retrieved April 3, 2010 from
http://www.helpguide.org/elder/picks_disease.htm

Hitti, M. (2006). FDA approves drug to treat Parkinson's dementia.
Retrieved March 31, 2010 from http://www.webmd.
com/parkinsons-disease/news/20060628/fda-oks-drug-
parkinsons-dementia

Mayo Clinic. (2010). Parkinson's disease. Retrieved March 31,
2010 from http://www.mayoclinic.com/health/parkinsons-
disease/DS00295

Mayo Clinic. (2010). Vascular Dementia. Retrieved March 31,
2010 from http://www.mayoclinic.com/health/vascular-
dementia/DS00934

MedicineNet. (2010). What is Dementia? Retrieved March 29,
2010 from http://www.medicinenet.com/dementia/page2.
htm

Medscape. (2001). Quetiapine Improves Symptoms of Parkinson's Disease. Retrieved April 2, 2010 from http://www.medscape.com/viewarticle/411260

Merck Manual. (2010). Dementia. Retrieved April 2, 2010 from http://www.merck.com/mmhe/sec06/ch083/ch083c.html#sec06-ch083-ch083c-541n

Pollock, B. (2007). SSRI Comparable to Antipsychotic for Psychosis in Dementia. American Journal of Geriatric Psychiatry. Retrieved April 2, 2010 from http://www.medpagetoday.com/Geriatrics/Dementia/6632

Swanberg, M. & Kalapatapu, R. (2010). Parkinson Disease Dementia: Treatment & Medication. Medscape. Retrieved April 2, 2010 from http://emedicine.medscape.com/article/289595-treatment

Chapter 5

Driving with Dementia, OH MY!

We all know it happens; individuals with dementia are often still driving in the early stage of their disease. Families and other caregivers worry about safety – both of the individual as well as the community in which they drive. This chapter will provide some insight into how dementia, as well as normal aging changes, affect driving abilities in elders. There will be a discussion of how driving is often viewed as a form of self-reliance and independence and how cessation of driving impacts an individual's life. Strategies will be presented to assist caregivers in stopping individuals from driving when it is no longer appropriate or safe.

Introduction

More than 5 million people in the United States are afflicted with dementia and a significant percentage of these individuals are still driving. Deciding when to limit or stop driving can be a confusing issue for individuals diagnosed with dementia as well as their families and caregivers. Since many times the diagnosis of dementia is being made earlier and medications are being used to slow its progression, there are many of these individuals driving longer than in previous years. This is presenting safety concerns as well as concerns about the person becoming lost and being unable to get back home. The main issue is when driving should cease and how to convince individuals with dementia that they should stop driving. Most information about dementia warns against driving. But many individuals with dementia may not realize the dangers and continue to drive. Most literature does not describe when or how to stop individuals driving who are cognitively impaired. The following discussion will assist in identifying the potential problems as well as provide suggestions for curbing or stopping driving (Hartford, 2010).

Driving Means Independence

Driving represents independence and control. It's a way to go and do what one wishes to do, when one wish to do it. It gives one the ability to go to stores – buy necessities, go to appointments – access healthcare, be productive, and stay connected to family, friends and the community. In the early stages of dementia, when individuals are still independent, is when families, as well as the individual with dementia, may begin to worry about when driving will no longer be safe. There are changes occurring in later life that affect driving in elders including vision problems, hearing deficits, and slower reaction times. And physical changes in older adults combined with the cognitive and mental changes occurring in individuals suffering from dementia can significantly affect the ability to drive. While most individuals continue to drive all of their lives, individuals with dementia will need to cease driving as their disease progresses.

Changes in Individuals with Dementia

The progression of dementia can differ according to the type of dementia from which an individual is suffering. In Alzheimer's disease the progression is usually gradual and somewhat predictable but will vary from one person to the next. Dementia affects cognitive functions which are critical to driving. Everyone with Alzheimer's disease or other irreversible dementias will have problems with:

- judgment
- multi-tasking
- slowed reaction times
- impaired spatial skills
- other cognitive deficits

(Hartford, 2010)

Dementia affects a person's capacity to assess driving abilities that may be diminished. This can be due to denial or an inability

96

to recognize the problem by a person and/or a spouse. People with dementia are likely to minimize the complexity of driving and overestimate their own abilities. They may make excuses for their high-risk driving behaviors, believing there is not a problem and that they are no different from other individuals their age.

Mom's Story

Mom used to say, 'all my friends forget a little, I am no different from them – there is nothing wrong with me.' Her driving abilities began to surface shortly after we realized there was a problem. I did notice multiple cigarette burns on her car seats as well as spilled drinks on the seats and floorboards. There were dents in the garage wall where she pulled in a little too close, there were marks on the tires from scrubbing the curbs too closely, there were small dents in the sides of the car, and well let's just say I felt really sorry for the mailbox (which was replaced repeatedly).

I had the chance to observe her driving and was surprised – she drove 20 miles under the speed limit, almost in the center of the road and would then jerk back into her own lane when oncoming traffic was close; she would stop 6 feet before the stop sign or in the middle of the intersection. There were definite safety concerns.

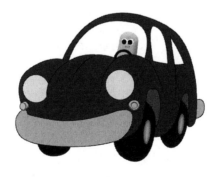

What are other risk factors for 'Normal' Elders & Driving?

While some elders are behind the wheel well into their eighth or ninth decade of life, some are not (or should not be) due to physical changes associated with aging which can make driving unsafe. Some key concerns which can affect elderly drivers include:

Physical Changes Which can Affect an Elder's Driving Abilities
*Not all elders will experience all of these changes but many will be affected by these common changes due to normal aging processes.

Vision: All elders experience some degree of decline in vision	• Depth perception: The cornea, the part of the eye which refracts light, becomes flatter, less smooth, and thicker making older eyes more susceptible to astigmatism. These changes can affect the ability to judge distance including judging the speed of oncoming traffic.
	• Decreased ability to differentiate colors: There is a yellowing of the lens which causes some reduction of the eye's ability to discriminate blues, greens, and violets; colors seen more clearly are yellows, oranges, and reds.
	• Ptosis: An older person may have loose skin on the lids of the eye. Eyelids may droop as elasticity is lost, causing the person's visual field to be diminished.
	• Dry Eyes: There can be a decrease in orbicular muscle strength causing the eyelid to stay open slightly which can lead to corneal dryness.
	• Presbyopia: After 40 years of age, a person's eye losses the ability to adjust to close objects and this problem continues to progress throughout life leading to a progressive farsightedness.
	• Decreased Peripheral Vision: Peripheral vision decreases making the visual field less (a person can no longer see things approaching from the side as readily).

Vision (continued)

- Slower Pupil Accommodation: Pupil size is smaller creating a slower constriction in the presence of bright light. There is a slowing of the pupil's dilation in dark settings and a slowing in the ability to accommodate to changes in light. Older eyes need three times more light, making night vision somewhat impaired in older adults. Glare occurs more often for elders. For example sunlight may be reflected off shiny objects or there may be a glare around headlights of other cars.

- Glaucoma: The anterior chamber of the eye decreases as the thickness of the lens increases. In some elders, there is an increase in the density of collagen fibers leading to inefficient resorption of intraocular fluids and increased pressure in the eye – glaucoma.

- Cataracts: Lens opacities can develop after the age of 50 causing cloudiness in vision and can progress to obscure vision completely. The vitreous humor, which gives the eye its shape and support, loses some of its fluid and fibrous support.

- Opacities can develop and can be seen as spots or clusters of dots in the visual field which are coalesced vitreous that have broken off the periphery or central part of the retina. These are largely harmless, although they can be annoying. Drusen (yellow-white) spots can develop in an area of the macula and, as long as not accompanied with distortion of objects or a decrease in vision, this pigmentation is not clinically significant.

continued on page 100

Hearing loss
Approximately 1/3 of elders have some degree of hearing impairment. It can occur gradually. A cue to a hearing problem when driving is inattention to sounds such as honking, emergency sirens, or a child's bicycle bell.

- Cerumen (Ear Wax): The Auditory canal narrows and the cerumen glands atrophy in older adults causing thicker and dryer cerumen (ear wax) which makes its removal more difficult and can lead to blockage of the canal.
- Presbycusis (Hearing Loss): The tympanic membrane becomes dull, less flexible, retracted, and slightly gray in appearance. The ossicle joints between the malleus and stapes can become calcified and lead to a reduction in vibration of these bones and thus reduced sound transmission. There is a slight degeneration of the internal parts of the ear which leads to impaired transmission of sound waves along the nerve pathways. These changes are considered the most common reason for hearing loss in elders. Another type of hearing loss is caused by atrophy of the organ of Corti which is sensory hearing loss. Loss of cochlear neurons can cause neural hearing loss.
- Tinnitis: Sometimes there is an impairment of the otic nerve which can lead to a constant or recurring high-pitched tinnitus such as clicking, buzzing, roaring, or ringing sound in one or both ears. Causes of this problem include medications, infections, or cerumen accumulation; a blow to the head can also cause this problem. Tinnitus can be more pronounced in quiet settings.

Motor skills **Full range of motion and good muscle strength are crucial for safety when an elder is on the road driving. Certain chronic conditions in elders can limit mobility. Illnesses such as rheumatoid arthritis, Parkinson's disease, sleep apnea, heart disease and diabetes can decrease flexibility and reaction time, raising the risks for accidents.**	• <u>Loss of Strength</u>: Muscles, tendons, and joints can lose some strength and flexibility with aging unless the elder is physically active. These changes can lead to a slower reaction time in response to stimuli. For example, an elder may need to stop quickly to avoid oncoming traffic but is unable to react rapidly enough to avoid an accident. • <u>Decreased Range of Motion of the Neck</u>: Bone mass or density can diminish as bones lose calcium and other minerals, especially in women after menopause. The spine is made up of several bones which have a gel-like cushion between them. In aging, the disks gradually lose fluid and become thinner causing the spinal column to become curved and compressed leading to kyphosis. Bone spurs can occur due to aging and overall use of the spine. The cumulative effect is decreased ability to turn one's head adequately to see oncoming traffic.
<u>Drowsiness</u> or sleepiness. Certain medications can cause drowsiness. Additionally, some elders become tired during the day or have an increased tendency to doze off during the day (or while driving).	• <u>Medications</u> that don't mix well with driving include: o benzodiazepines o some antihistamines o certain glaucoma medications o non-steroidal anti-inflammatory drugs o muscle relaxants

(Aging Eyes 2006; Ebersole et al, 2004; Eye Digest, 2010; MedicineNet, 2006; Helpguide's Senior Driving: Risk Factors, Safety Tips and Transportation Options; Tumosa, 2000)

Driving with Dementia

A diagnosis of dementia is not automatically a reason to take away driving privileges. There is no examination and no single indicator to determine when an individual with dementia poses a danger to self or others when driving. Individuals suffering from dementia and their families must determine when an individual is unsafe to drive. Some key indicators which provide clues that a person's driving abilities may not be safe include:

- Poor attention span
- Inability to judge distance
- Inability to process information making difficult to respond safely in driving situations

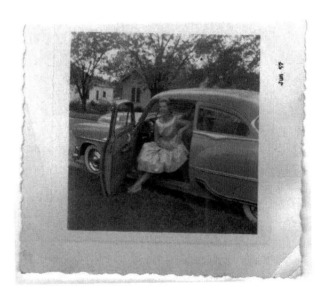

Warning Signs for Drivers with Dementia

Riding the brake

Easily distracted while driving

Other drivers often honk horns

Incorrect signaling

Difficulty parking within a defined space

Hitting curbs or other cars

Scrapes or dents on the car, mailbox, or garage

Increased agitation or irritation when driving

Failure to notice activity on the side of the road

Failure to follow instructions on traffic signs (or even notice them) i.e., speed limits, yield signs, 'do not enter', 'one way'

Trouble navigating complex situations

Driving at inappropriate speeds – either too slow or too fast

Not anticipating potentially dangerous situations

Uses a copilot

Bad judgment when making turns

Close calls or near accidents

Slow or delayed response to unexpected situations

Drifting into the wrong lane

Difficulty maintaining lane position

Confusion at entrances or exits

Moving violation tickets or warnings

Getting lost in familiar places

Car accidents

Failure to stop at stop sign or red light

Confusing the gas and brake pedals

Stopping in traffic for no apparent reason

(Hartford, 2010)

Weighing the Risks (Safety) against the Benefits (an Individual's Independence & Autonomy) of Driving

Safety trumps autonomy when circumstances are evident that elders and others are at risk (or in danger) due to the effects an individual's dementia upon their driving abilities. But when the threat is not absolutely clear to an individual that there is a significant problem and the family's wishes (the person not drive due to safety concerns) differ from the individual's wishes (to continue to drive based on a desire for autonomy, independence, and control), conflict is inevitable. Moreover the consequences to the older person of giving up driving are not trivial and the burdens imposed by loss of the driving privileges, as well as loss of independence, are both practical and psychological. For individuals who may be isolated from others, whether living in rural or suburban environments, a personal automobile may be the only readily available means of transportation. In urban areas there may be public transportation, taxi or car services available but many elders are not familiar with using this type of transportation and may find it confusing. Relaying on others for transportation is not always a welcome solution for many elders even if it is provided by family or friends. Convincing an older individual with a diagnosis of dementia to retire from driving for 'safety's sake' will sometimes have undesirable consequences including rebellion by an elder or an argument (Kennedy, 2009).

Use the **Warning Signs for Drivers with Dementia** to help families and caregivers better understand when an individual's ability to drive is becoming unsafe and there is decline in an individual's abilities as the disease progresses.

- Consider the frequency and severity of incidents
  - Several minor incidents or an unusual, major incident may require immediate action
- Look for patterns of change over time
  - Isolated or minor incidents may not require immediate or drastic action

- Avoid an alarming reaction
  - Take notes and have conversations at a later, convenient time

Share observations with the individual who has a diagnosis of dementia, family members, and caregivers. Families need to consider the circumstances and seriousness of unsafe driving practices before deciding the next steps which should be taken – choices include:

1. continue monitoring
2. modify driving
3. stop driving immediately

How is an Elder Driver Evaluated when Safety is a Concern?

When there is suspicion that an individual might be an unsafe driver, close monitoring is essential before a definitive decision should be made, whether it is time to limit driving or give up the driver's license altogether. Some steps include:

- Watch for changes in driving habits, general behavior, and any other health issues which could affect driving
- Encourage a driving evaluation through the local Department of Motor Vehicles, along with refresher driving lessons. AARP encourages a "Driver Safety course" for elders who are having problems with driving
- Reduce the need to drive
  - have family or friends pick up the individual to go shopping or to go out for dinner
  - home delivery or services provided at home
    - » shop online and through mail order catalogues
    - » have necessities delivered – groceries, medications, or meals

>> have others make home visits to the person when possible – clergy, medical and personal care providers

>> arrange for a barber or hairdresser to make home visits

>> schedule people to visit regularly, either as volunteers or for pay

- If necessary, obtain support from the person's healthcare provider and other family members

Easing the Transition from Driving

One of the most difficult tasks for families to accomplish is transitioning an individual from driving. But family members must balance the needs and safety of their loved ones against the safety of the community in which they live. Any person who takes on the task of 'taking the keys away' may be considered the the bad guy or 'black sheep' of the family, not just for a day or two, but for a long time. This person may be the one upon whom the burden of care resides when the individual needs anything or wishes to go anywhere.

Mom's Rebellion When the Keys were Taken

When it was time to take Mom's keys away, Mom and I discussed the issues revolving around safety of driving and the incidents which were making me come to this decision. Mom did not see the need to stop driving but I did. When the time came, I was called names I didn't even know she knew. I was called at 2 a.m. when she was out of cigarettes or needed milk.

Beginning the Process of Stopping a Person (with Dementia) from Driving

The most effective approach to limit or stop a person from driving involves developing a plan and will probably include a combination of strategies that fit the circumstances, resources, and relationships. For individuals in the early stages of dementia, it may be a better approach to reduce the person's frequency of driving over time rather than stopping it abruptly. Attention should be given to meeting a person's day-to-day needs including obtaining food, medications, and medical needs. It is also important to address a person's social needs. Whenever possible, include the person with dementia in planning ahead to limit and eventually stop driving.

Fortunately, in many cases, individuals with dementia often realize there may be a problem and begin limiting where and when they drive. Some individuals who choose to limit their own driving attribute the reason to physical complaints. The following signs indicate that a person with dementia is modifying their driving behaviors:

- Drives only short distances
- Drives only to familiar places
- Avoids difficult situations
- Avoids driving at night, in heavy traffic, on heavily traveled roads and/or during bad weather

Keep in mind that driving even short distances during daylight hours and in good weather can pose a risk if one's driving skills are impaired. Most accidents have been reported to occur close to home (Hartford, 2010).

Enough is Enough; Driving MUST be Stopped

Sometimes an individual with a diagnosis of dementia has to be 'stopped' from driving over his/her objections. It might be very difficult for families to come to this decision, especially if the individual is very independent. However, the safety of the person and the safety of others must come first. An unsafe driver can seriously injure or kill themselves or others.

If appropriate evaluations and recommendations have been made, driving is no longer safe, and rational discussions with the person have not been successful in persuading a person to stop driving, then creativity in finding a solution is a necessity. This can be a difficult task and each situation requires an individualized plan. In some cases, there is a need to take further actions such as taking away the car keys, selling or disabling the vehicle, and/or enlisting authority figures including healthcare providers or the local police to assist in explaining the importance of safe driving and the legal implications of unsafe driving (HelpGuide, 2010).

Legal Restrictions for Elder Drivers

A person's age is not a sufficient basis for losing a driver's license or even for a person to be mandated to undergo re-examination for a driver's license. Older individuals do not automatically lose their driving privileges and/or drivers licenses with a diagnosis of dementia because they have certain legal rights. State Departments of Motor Vehicles (DMV) do have the authority to investigate and re-examine any individual who demonstrates a potential risk of driving dangerously due to physical, psychiatric, or behavioral problems or there is evidence of poor driving record.

State-by-state Regulations on Elderly Drivers License Renewal

- Six states (Florida, Maine, Oregon, South Carolina, Utah, and Virginia) and the District of Columbia require elderly drivers to take a vision test when renewing a license
- Another way states monitor older drivers is by no longer permitting drivers over a certain age to renew their licenses by mail
  - Five states (Alaska, California, Colorado, Louisiana, and Montana) restrict mail renewals and online renewal
  - Finally, two states (Illinois and New Hampshire) require a road test if the driver is 75 years old or older

State Legal Requirements to Report an Unsafe Driver

- All state Departments of Motor Vehicles, Highway Safety, or Transportation have an office where a family member or healthcare provider can make a referral about an unsafe driver
  - The state DMV office will investigate the claim to determine if the driver should be mandated to take a road test in order to maintain his/her license
- In California, however, healthcare providers are required to submit a confidential report of individuals who have a diagnosis of dementia

'This information is forwarded to the Department of Motor Vehicles (DMV), which is authorized to take action against the driving privileges of any individual who is unable to safely operate a motor vehicle. If the physician's report indicates that an individual has *moderate* or *severe* dementia, that individual will no longer be permitted to operate a motor vehicle. DMV has determined that *only drivers with dementia in the mild stages may still have the cognitive functions necessary to continue driving safely.* DMV requires re-examination for all individuals reported to have mild dementia.'

Family Caregiver Alliance, (2010)

  - Compared to other medical issues which affect driving abilities: In California, Delaware, Nevada, New Jersey, Oregon, and Pennsylvania, healthcare providers are required to report individuals with a diagnosis of epilepsy

California DMV Procedure in Management of Individuals with Dementia

The California DMV follows specific procedures when a medical report regarding an individual with dementia is received:

1. A computer search is conducted to locate the individual's name, verify that he/she has a license, and examine the driving history
2. The individual is contacted by letter and sent a "Driver Medical Evaluation" form to authorize the primary healthcare provider to submit medical information about the status of the dementia including the person's cognitive functioning
3. A Driver Safety hearing officer reviews the medical form: If the person is in the mild stage of dementia, the individual is scheduled for a re-examination with DMV; if the individual is in the later stages of dementia, their driving privileges will be revoked; and if the individual fails to submit medical documentation within the requested time frame, all driving privileges will be suspended.
4. A re-examination is completed, involving three phases: a **visual test**, a **written test**, and an **interview**.
   - **Visual Test**: Effective January 1, 2001, all drivers must have corrected visual acuity of better than 20/200 in the better eye without the use of a bioptic telescope
   - **Written Test**: The individual is given the standard DMV written examination designed to test an individual's knowledge of the road. The written test allows the DMV office to determine not only the person's knowledge of driving laws, but also mental competency and cognitive skills
   - **Interview**: An in-person interview focuses on the medical documentation as well as the driver's ability to coherently answer questions about his/her health, medical treatment, driving record, need to drive, daily routine, need for assistance with daily activities, etc. Persons who do well

up to this point are then given a driving test. Those who do poorly on the visual, written, or verbal tests may have their driving privilege suspended or revoked.

5. The driving test is designed to test driving skills that might be affected by dementia.
   - Initially, the person is observed to identify if the individual can find his/her car. Then, the examiner gives a series of commands, rather than one direction at a time (for example, "Please drive to the corner, turn left and turn right at the first street"). The test generally lasts longer than the ordinary driver's test in order to gauge whether or not fatigue is a problem.

6. If the individual passes the driving test, the license is generally not suspended or revoked although restrictions may be imposed on the license, such as no freeway driving, no night driving, or driving allowed only within a certain radius. DMV may want to review the individual's driving skills again in six to twelve months. At that time the entire process begins again.

7. An appeals process is available if the individual or family wishes to contest the suspension or revocation of the driver's license. At the hearing the individual may present evidence, such as new medical information, to prove that the dementia does not impair his or her ability to safely operate a motor vehicle.

8. DMV can provide a California identification card to those persons who will no longer have a driver's license.

(Family Caregiver Alliance, 2010)

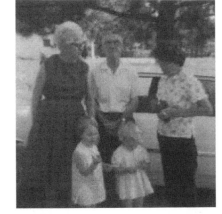

111

Steps to 'Taking the Keys' and Stopping Driving

1. **Identify the Problem: It begins with admitting an Individual's driving is an issue**
   - ❖ **Assess an Individual's driving abilities**
   - ❖ **Ride along and observe**
   - ❖ **Have a friend or another relative ride along and observe**
   - ❖ **Have the Person meet a third party who can observe the person's driving abilities:**
     - » Make sure the observer arrives prior to the person who is being evaluated
     - » The observer should be positioned in order to watch the driver's arrival
     - » Make sure to have the person navigate an intersection – preferably a stop sign – have the person cross/turn at a stop sign
     - » Watch for use of blinkers
     - » Watch for appropriateness of stopping – Problems: Stopping too far back from line or in middle of intersection
     - » Watch ability in crossing intersection with other traffic – Problems: hesitation to enter intersection or entering intersection out of turn
     - » Watch the person park – Problems: parking too close to other vehicles, parking too far into space or too far back

     REMEMBER SAFETY: Time of day – avoid evening and night-time, light traffic times, and good weather
2. **Identify State laws and restrictions on Individual Drivers as well as Drivers with a diagnosis of dementia**
3. **Enlist the Individual Driver in discussions about stopping driving**

4. Keep a driving log to document problems

* Drives too slowly
* Stops in traffic for no reason or ignores traffic signs
* Becomes lost on a familiar route
* Lacks good judgment
* Has difficulty with turns, lane changes, or highway exits
* Drifts into other lanes of traffic or drives on the wrong side of the street
* Signals incorrectly or does not signal
* Has difficult seeing pedestrians, objects, or other vehicles
* Falls asleep while driving or gets drowsy
* Parks inappropriately
* Gets ticketed for traffic violations
* Is increasingly nervous or irritated when driving
* Has accidents, near misses, or "fender benders"

5. Decrease the person's need to drive and/or limit driving

* Have groceries, meals, and prescriptions delivered to the home
* Arrange for a barber or hairdresser to make home visits – or – go to hairdresser together
* Invite friends and family over for regular visits
* Arrange for family and friends to take the individual on social outings

6. When the time comes for the person to stop driving: Discuss your observations with the person – use the driving log – the list of reasons why the person is not safe to continue driving; if the discussion becomes heated, this will assist in your ability to make your points

continued on page 114

7. **Suggestions for stopping a person from driving, if persuasion fails, include:**
   - ❖ Hiding the car keys
   - ❖ Replacing the car keys with a set that won't start the car (men figure this one out rather more quickly)
   - ❖ Disabling or selling the car
   - ❖ Moving the car out of sight (remember to notify local police so when the person calls to report the car stolen, they are aware of the issues)

Taking Mom's Keys

Mom's driving was pretty bad – she went very slow, stopped 4-5 feet before stop signs and didn't alternate well with other traffic; she would veer toward the center lane and often see oncoming traffic and almost swerve into the ditch on the side of the road; had multiple dents in the car as well as on the poor wall in her garage; there were no more hub caps on the wheels; and the problem was apparent. I tried to do a ride-along to observe her driving abilities but she said she did not do well because I made her nervous and she knew I was checking things out. So I asked a friend of hers to do a ride-along (her brave friend), well – friends are really going to be pulling for the person because they are also in this age group and they want the person to do well, but her friend admitted there were issues. So I had her meet me for a late lunch and waited where I could see her coming. I arrived early (didn't want to miss her arrival), sat near a window, and had her meet me where she had to navigate a stop sign (not a light – if it were green, I wouldn't have seen anything). It really validated my concerns about the driving problem. So we had to figure out a way to take the keys away and stop her from driving. Next, we had to develop a plan.

Alternatives to Driving

Asking an individual to stop driving can be a delicate issue. Be prepared when the person asks how they will get around or get the things they need. Have a plan and the appropriate answers prepared.

Let Others Do the Driving – explore all transportation options – from public transportation to informal arrangements with families, friends, and support groups.

Public Transportation – an option if the individual can maneuver this type of transportation and it is accessible to the person. But this type of transportation can be extremely complicated for individuals with moderate to advanced dementia.

Pay-for-service Transportation – Taxis can be a cost-effective alternative, especially when fares are compared to the expense of gas, insurance, taxes, repairs and car payments. Taxis could be used for people in middle to later stages of dementia if:

• There are no behavioral problems and the driver can be given explicit directions
• In the moderate to advanced stages of dementia, someone may need to be available to meet the person at the beginning and end of the trip

*Some taxi companies will set up accounts for family caregivers so a person with dementia has easy access to transportation without worrying about payment.

Friends and Relatives or caregivers can offer to drive the individual with dementia to appointments or other social events. Families will be more likely to assist with driving if the primary caregiver makes specific requests and schedules appointments at times that work for those requested to help.

Co-Piloting Is <u>Not</u> a Good Solution – Some families or caregivers act as co-pilots to keep an individual with dementia driving longer, giving directions and instructions on how to drive. Although this strategy may work for a limited time, it can be hazardous and there is rarely enough time for a driver suffering from dementia to foresee the danger and respond quickly enough to avoid an accident.

Early Planning to Limit Driving

When possible, include the individual with dementia in discussions surrounding driving safety and future plans to cease driving. It is better to obtain the person's input and understand their point of view while conveying how dementia will eventually affect the person's ability to drive. It is better to convey to a person the reasons, while the person can still understand these reasons, why this decision will be necessary, and allow the person to understand the rational arguments for safety. This method respects the individual's dignity by focusing on how the disease affects the person, not that the individual is any lesser a person, as the reason for driving restrictions and cessation.

Build Social Support to reduce stress and increase chances for success. Encourage the person to increase the use of others to meet the needs the person would normally meet through driving. Relying on others for emotional support, transportation assistance, and financial help or to meet other needs are good alternatives. For example, a child or neighbor might be able to run an errand or pay a visit; a long-distance relative might be willing to pay for an occasional driver or taxi; or a friend might be able to observe driving ability and habits.

Other Opportunities to Limit Driving

With some foresight and planning, families may be able to create non-confrontational ways to make driving less appealing or less necessary. Some examples include:

- When an individual with a diagnosis of dementia is moving to an area that has more support services, discuss alternative transportation in the new location – particularly because these individuals may be more uncomfortable and at higher risk of accidents when driving in unfamiliar places (Relocation may help encourage the individual to limit or stop driving).
- Families may be able to use discussions surrounding financial issues to build a case for selling the car by itemizing the many costs of operating a vehicle including upkeep, taxes, tag, gasoline, and insurance costs.
- Physical changes which affect driving may be used as an excuse to limit or stop driving (see physical changes listed earlier in this chapter).

Taking the Keys should be the Last Resort BUT may be Necessary

Taking away the keys or a person's driver's license as well as selling or disabling a person's car should only be done as a last resort. To an individual in the early stages of dementia, such actions can seem extreme, disrespectful, and punitive. And people in the later stages of dementia can ignore requests to stop driving, drive without a license, or forget they have been told to stop driving. When steps have been taken to make the car inaccessible such as a car being 'disabled', they have someone 'fix' the problem or when they cannot locate their car, they replace the car with another vehicle. Once an individual with dementia has stopped driving, families must decide whether taking away the keys, license, and car will help the person adjust or make it more difficult.

Mom's Revolt when the Keys were Taken

We had begun talking to Mom about her driving and how she might be having problems but Mom said she didn't drive much and only drove when she needed something. In observing her abilities, it became apparent continued driving was not a safe option for her or the community in which she lived. The time came to take the keys. We discussed the problem, and against her wishes, I took her keys. Mom actually had 6 sets of keys – she had multiple sets made because she would misplace them frequently. After I took the last set, she had a friend help her figure out how to have another set made – they obtained the Vehicle Identification Number – VIN from the vehicle and called the dealership to have a new set of keys made, then had someone pick them up for her. Now, I began to ponder, if she was that ingenious to figure a way out to get another set of keys, maybe she could continue driving. BUT I knew better; I had observed her driving abilities and it was not safe.

The next step was to disable the car – I told her when we got enough money, we would consider having it fixed (to avoid another argument). The first time we disabled it, my niece's boyfriend fixed it. So we told all the close family members not to 'fix' her car. The second time we disabled the car, a neighbor fixed it. We then told near-by neighbors to please not help 'fix' the car.

We did finally manage to stop Mom's driving; she lived a few minutes from me because she wished to remain independent. We made arrangements and took turns going by daily to check on her. We would call to check on her during the daytime as well as made sure Mom had all of our numbers on speed dial in case she needed anything. I would take her shopping weekly as well as get her anything she needed. One of us would take her to church services and any appointments to which she needed to go. Of course, it was not easy at first. She was very angry, called me nasty names and would call me at all hours when she thought of something she needed. But it was in her best interest and, out of love, we took the things she said and did in stride. This lasted a few months before she finally got over the anger and frustration.

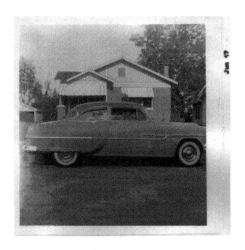

Chapter 5 References

Aging Eyes (2006). Retrieved April 4, 2010 from http://agingeye.net

Dobbs, A. R. (1997). "Evaluating the Driving Competence of Dementia Patients." *Alzheimer's Disease and Associated Dementia.* Vol. 11, Suppl: 8-12.

Ebersole, Hess, & Luggen (2004). Toward Healthy Aging. 6th ed. Mosby, Inc: Philadelphia.

Family Caregiver Alliance. (2010). Dementia, Driving, and California State Law. Retrieved April 4, 2010 from http://www.caregiver.org/caregiver/jsp/content_node.jsp?nodeid=433

Hartford Foundation (2000). At the Crossroads: A Guide to Alzheimer's Disease, Dementia, and Driving. From www.thehartford.com/alzheimers

Hartford Foundation. (2010). Family discussions about Alzheimer's disease, dementia, and driving. Retrieved April 2, 2010 from http://www.thehartford.com/alzheimers

HelpGuide. (2010). Helpguide's Senior Driving: Risk Factors, Safety Tips and Transportation Options. Retrieved April 4, 2010 from http://beta.helpguide.org/elder/senior_citizen_driving.htm

Kennedy, G. (2009). Psychogeriatrics: Advanced Age, Dementia, and Driving. *Psychiatric Weekly.* 4(18). Retrieved April 3, 2010 from http://www.psychiatryweekly.com/aspx/article/articledetail.aspx?articleid=984

LA 4 Seniors.com (2001). *Dangerous Driving and Seniors.* from www.la4seniors.com/driving.htm

Mayo Foundation for Medical Education and Research (2001). *Dementia: Should Your Patient be Driving?* from www.mayo.edu/geriatrics-rst/driving.html

MedicineNet (2006). Hearing loss and aging. Retrieved October
14, 2006 from http://www.medicinenet.com/script/main/art.
asp?articlekey=20432

Tumosa, N. (2000). Aging and the eye. *Merck manual of geriatrics*.
Whitehouse Station, NJ. Merck research Laboratories.

Chapter 6

Sundowning, Wandering, and Aggressive Behaviors (Physical Aggression & Sexually Inappropriate Behaviors)

This chapter will include a brief discussion of 'Sundowning' and why it can occur in elders. Common problematic behaviors reported in individuals suffering from dementia will be presented including examples of triggers which may be causing the behavior to occur. Strategies to diminish the occurrence of behaviors as well as ways to manage behaviors will be reviewed, a brief discussion on why orientation theory is 'out-the-door', and the importance of validation and redirection – many examples of techniques will be reviewed including ways to decrease the bathing battle.

Introduction

Thoughts, emotions, personality, and behaviors can be affected by cognitive impairment. Dementias, including those caused by Alzheimer's disease, affect the brain and affect what a person thinks, feels, and how emotions are expressed – essentially how a person behaves and a individual's basic personality. Alzheimer's disease, the most common cause of dementia in older adults, affects various parts of the brain at different times and advances at different rates in each person with the disease, making it hard to predict how a person will behave.

Personality traits of individuals suffering from dementia may become more exaggerated – the usual personality more pronounced, for example individuals who were concerned with money become obsessed with it or individuals who were often worried become constant worriers. Or the person's personality becomes opposite from the person's usual demeanor, for example individuals who were once quiet become verbally and/or physically aggressive or a person who was very outspoken all his life becomes withdrawn and no longer talkative. Some individuals become irritable, anxious, self-centered, inflexible, or more easily angered while others become more passive, expressionless, depressed, indecisive, or withdrawn. If changes in behavior are brought to the person's attention, he/she may become hostile or agitated (Merck, 2010). Dementia makes it more difficult for an individual to remember things, think clearly, communicate with others, or take care of him/herself. It may even cause mood swings. Each person will present with different behaviors and personalities which will require an individualized management strategy to optimize care.

Key Things to Remember in Communicating with Individuals Suffering from Dementia

Improving communication skills will diminish the incidence of certain behavioral problems which arise in individuals suffering from dementia as well as assist in managing these problems. Good communication can create an environment that is less stressful and will likely improve the quality of life for these individuals. The following suggestions will also enhance a caregiver's ability to handle day-to-day life.

1. **Set a positive mood for interaction.** Pay careful attention to mannerisms, attitude, and body language – the person's as well as the caregiver's. Set a positive mood by speaking in a pleasant and respectful manner. Use simplistic words but not 'baby' talk. Use facial expressions, an even tone of voice, and physical touch to help maintain a humanistic relationship with the person as well as convey messages. When an individual is agitated and behaving aggressively, speak to the person in an even monotone voice with a matter-of-fact tone and do not tense up with aggressive or defensive body language (agitated individuals usually react to the response they receive e.g., if the caregiver responds as with surprise and an upset manner, the person may become more defensive and upset, further escalating the problem.)

2. **Get the person's attention.** Limit distractions and noise – it may be helpful to turn off background noise from a radio or television, close the curtains or shut the door, or consider moving to quieter area when trying to communicate or accomplish a task with the person. Address a person by name, identify yourself by name and relation, and use nonverbal cues such as hand signals or attempt to demonstrate the action the caregiver wishes the person to emulate. Consider using touch to keep the person engaged and help keep the person focused. Speak according to the person's educational level, maintain eye contact, and if possible do not stand in a dominating position, since standing over a person may make the person feel threatened – such as when the person is seated and the caregiver is standing to the side and looking down at the person.

3. **Use simple words, concrete terms, and short single sentences.** Attention should be given to using terminology that is simplistic and concrete. Sentences should be short and concise so the person can follow a train of thought or an instruction. When a lengthy discussion, a long explanation, or a series of instructions are given, the person may become lost due to memory impairment and not being able to remember the first part of what they are being told. Instructions should be given one at a time and the person allowed to complete one step before another instruction is given, since the person may forget the first instruction when trying to concentrate on the next instruction being given. Abstract words may not be understood or may be confused with a concrete definition. For example do not say 'hop on the bed', the person may not understand that the caregiver intends the person to sit on the bed – it would be more appropriate to simply say 'please sit on the bed'.

4. **Make speech heard more clearly.** Speak slowly, distinctly and in a reassuring tone but refrain from raising the tone of

voice that is either higher or louder. Instead attempt to lower the voice pitch of your voice to make the words more easily heard by an older individual who may have some degree of hearing loss.

5. **Ask simple, answerable questions.** Ask one question at a time and refrain from asking open-ended questions such as 'What would you like to eat?' Also, do not give a person too many choices or the person may be overwhelmed and not able to make a decision at all. It is better to ask questions which offer limited choices such as 'Would you like to eat a hamburger or a salad?' Make efforts not to ask questions that can be answered with yes or no response such as 'Do you need to use the bathroom?' Instead ask leading questions such as 'Let's go try to use the bathroom, okay?'

6. **Break down activities into a series of steps.** Offer one instruction at a time and allow the person to complete the requested task before offering another instruction. This makes many tasks much more manageable. Encourage the person to do what he/she is able to do, gently remind the person of steps that are forgotten, and assist with steps a person is no longer able to accomplish without assistance. Use visual cues, such as pointing to where the person should sit, demonstrating how to put toothpaste on a toothbrush, etc.

7. **When the going gets tough, distract and redirect.** When a person becomes upset, attempt to redirect the person's attention away from why they are angry to calm an agitated or aggressive problem. Try talking about something else, changing the subject or the environment; for instance, talk about the weather or what the person is wearing, or encourage the person to do another task such as 'Let's go see what you would like to wear tomorrow,' or 'I wonder where Martha is, let's go see if we can find her.'

(Caregiver.org, 2010)

Why Problematic Behaviors Occur

It is important to remember that a person with a diagnosis of dementia has a physiological disease which can be expressed as behavioral problems including aggression, agitation, apathy, repetitive behaviors, suspicion, and wandering as well as 'sundowning' behaviors – increase in problematic behaviors in the afternoon, evening, and night-time hours (Alzheimer's Association, 2010). Behavioral and psychological symptoms may result from several functional changes related to dementia including:

- Reduced impulse control and reduced inhibition
- Misinterpretation of visual and auditory cues
- Impaired short-term memory
- Reduced ability (or inability) to express needs
- Poor ability to adapt to the regimentation of institutional living such as scheduled mealtimes, bedtimes, and toileting times that are not individualized
- Physical problems such as pain, shortness of breath, urinary retention, or constipation
- Depression may coincide with dementia. (Depression can be expressed as an abrupt change in cognition, decreased appetite, deterioration in mood, a change in sleep pattern – often hypersomnolence, withdrawal, decreased activity level, crying spells, talk of death and dying, sudden development of irritability or psychosis, or other sudden changes in behavior.)
- Psychotic behaviors such as the occurrence of delusions or hallucinations

(Merck Manual, 2010)

Lack of Control

Individuals suffering from dementia are less capable of controlling their behaviors and can act inappropriately or disruptively at times. These actions can be problematic when a person is unable to be reasoned with using a logical explanation because the person's

127

reasoning abilities are declining and sometimes behaviors escalate when the person is corrected. There are several reasons why dementia is problematic to manage and factors which contribute to the problem include:

- Because the person has forgotten the rules of proper behavior, the individual acts in a socially inappropriate way. For example when they are hot, some individuals may undress in public. When they have sexual impulses, some persons may masturbate in public, use off-color or lewd language, or make sexual demands.
- Because individuals with dementia may have difficulty interpreting what they see and hear or feel threatened and lash out. For example, when someone tries to help the person undress, they may interpret this as an invasion and try to protect themselves, sometimes becoming combative.
- Because short-term memory is impaired, some of these individuals cannot remember what they are being told or what they have done. They repeat questions and conversations, demand constant attention, or ask for things repeatedly. They may become agitated and upset when they do not receive answers to questions or get what they ask for.
- Because a person cannot express his/her needs clearly or at all, discomfort such as constipation, pain, or being hot/cold can cause the person to cry, yell, or wander. Or these behaviors can occur when the person is lonely or frightened.

Disinhibition

Many problematic behaviors can be exhibited by individuals suffering from dementia due to a lack of impulse control or **disinhibition** – a lack of social skills and restraint to adhere to social norms – which can be manifested in several ways, including disregard for acceptable behaviors, poor risk assessment, and impulsivity. For example a thought comes to mind and the person immediately says the thought without regard to who can hear or how the person says the idea, or a person is irritated by another individual and the disinhibited person hits the person who has irritated him. An individual suffering from dementia is less able to exercise normal control: to choose to inhibit some responses in the way most people would do each day for reasons of politeness, sensitivity, social appropriateness, or desire to keep our true feelings hidden from others (Wikipedia, 2010).

Disinhibition can be manifested as **hypersexuality** – being preoccupied with fondling self or others; **hyperphagia** – constantly eating or placing things in mouth; and aggressive outbursts – yelling, hitting, or other aggressive tendencies. An individual exhibiting disinhibiting behaviors is more prone to react according to feelings brought on by stimulation, time of day, degree of energy, or degree of fatigue. A person's reaction to stimuli may differ from one day to the next making behavior unpredictable.

Reasons for Disinhibiting Behaviors in Persons with Dementia

- Difficulty remembering social norms and rules of etiquette
- Difficulty remembering the consequences of a behavior
- Acting on impulse
- Poor abstract thinking
- Poor social judgment
- Being unable to express feelings or communicate in an appropriate way
- Misinterpreting social cues
  - interpreting someone's politeness as permission for touching or acceptance of flirting behaviors

Continued on page 130

- Response to factors in the environment
  - an elderly man might interpret activities such as cleaning when soiled from urine or feces – having his legs touched in order to clean or being given a bath by a young female caregiver (who does not provide an explanation prior to performing the activity) as a sexual advance from the caregiver
- Not understanding what they are being told
- Not comprehending the meaning of the words spoken to them
- Being confused about where the person is (thinking he or she is in the bathroom and starting to undress)
- Being confused by who the person is interacting with, such as caregivers and nursing home staff being confused with the person's wife or girlfriend
- Feeling lonely which can lead to repetitive behaviors, crying, or agitation
- Feelings of discomfort, such as being too hot or cold, may lead to undressing
- Urinary incontinence or a urinary tract infection may lead to sexual behaviors such as touching one's own genitals
- Constipation or being soiled from urinary or fecal incontinence may cause agitation

Inability to Interpret what a Person is Feeling or Needing; Inability to Express Self

Individuals suffering from dementia may not be able to understand certain feelings or sensations that they are experiencing. They may also have problems trying to express themselves. The following are issues which can occur when a person is having problems with misinterpretation:

- **Aphasia** – an acquired disturbance of language, an inability to form the word(s) the person is trying to say; for example using words that rhyme such as 'I am going to get my boat' instead of

'I am going to get my coat' or using a totally different word such as 'I am going to get my blurber.'

- **Apraxia** – an inability to order routine motor tasks; for example, the person is unable to comb hair or dress self, in an organized way.

- **Agnosia** – an inability to interpret sensory information despite not having a primary sensory deficit; for example, the person recognizes a fork but is unable to recognize what a fork is to be used for.

- **Problems with executive functioning** – exhibits poor judgment, is unable to process complex reasoning, has an inability to organize tasks, and has poor insight such as the person may believe that when a television commercial says 'You have won a million dollars,' the person believes he has really won a million dollars.

(APA-DSM TR-IV)

Acceptance of the Cause of Problematic Behaviors

The key to managing challenging behaviors in individuals suffering from dementia is to develop an understanding of the cause of the behaviors. It is a physiological disease affecting a person's brain leading to cognitive impairment and behavioral issues. Next accept the fact that some behaviors are a manifestation of the disease and not the person's intentional actions. And then view the behaviors through a compassionate, non-judgmental lens. To assist in managing problematic behaviors, try to identify any precursors which commonly occur when such behaviors are displayed. Begin by dissecting events occurring before, during, and after a behavior: Before – attempt to identify the cause of the behavior, such as any event that happens before a problematic behavior occurs, or commonly 'sets the stage' for problematic behavior(s) such as bath time causing a person to become upset; During – what is the behavior trying to express, for example irritation, discomfort, or a need like hunger, thirst, constipation, pain, or irritation such as the person becomes agitated when wet from urinary incontinence; and After – what are the consequences of the behavior each time the behavior occurs, for example attention or scolding – the person is given more attention when he/she cries (Hill, 2008).

Dissecting Problematic Behaviors: Before, During, & After

Before:

Does the person always become agitated after talking with a particular person?

Is he calm at home, but wanders when he's in a chaotic place like the grocery store?

Does she start moving repetitively before mealtimes?

Does he become aggressive immediately before a urinary incontinent episode?

Does she become more withdrawn when constipated?

During:

Is the person aggressive and the problem escalates when corrected?

Does he wander around looking for someone or something; wandering worsens when he is unable go where he wants to go?

Does she ask repetitive questions and no one provides an answer?

Does he scratch himself when no one is paying him any attention?

Does she spit, curse, or play in feces when bored?

After:

How does a caregiver react after the behavior occurs – anxious, upset, consoling, or ignore the person?

Do caregivers stay calm?

Does the caregiver become defensive?

Does the caregiver yell at the person?

Does the caregiver give the person more attention?

Troubling Behaviors Exhibited by Individuals with Dementia

- Pacing
- Inappropriate robing or disrobing
- Spitting
- Cursing
- Verbal aggression
- Constant hitting
- Kicking
- Grabbing
- Pushing
- Making strange noises
- Screaming
- Scratching
- Trying to get to a different place
- General restlessness
- Complaining
- Negativism
- Handling things inappropriately
- Hiding things
- Hoarding things
- Tearing things
- Performing repetitious mannerisms
- Verbal sexual advances
- Physical sexual advances
- Intentional falling
- Throwing things
- Biting
- Eating inappropriate substances
- Hurting oneself or others

(Guay & Lott, 2010)

Figure 11: Troubling Behaviors Exhibitied by Individuals with Dementia

Remember, individuals with a diagnosis of dementia cannot control or prevent behaviors on their own. It's up to caregivers to attempt to change the person's behavior by changing what happens before or after the behavior occurs in order to manage it more appropriately. AND change the way the caregiver responds to behaviors when they do occur.

(Hill, 2008)

Planning Care

Dementias are permanent conditions and progressive in nature. Planning for the future is essential when caring for individuals suffering from a disorder which causes a person to become demented. Decisions about moving an individual to a more supportive environment, such as a Nursing Home, will involve balancing the desire to keep a person safe with the desire to maintain the person's sense of independence. Staying in the home environment is optimal for most individuals to maintain routine and a sense of normalcy. It is often encouraged to maintain a person in their usual living environment for as long as possible. But safety and the person's well-being are major factors which necessitate a change and require placement in a more structured environment. Such decisions depend on many factors, including:

- Severity of the person's dementia
- How disruptive the person's behavior is
- Home environment & Safety factors
- Availability of family members and caregivers
- Financial resources
- Presence of other, unrelated disorders and physical problems

Principles for Management of Behavioral
Problems in Individuals with Dementia

- Acceptance of the person
- Non-confrontational interactions
- Maintain optimal autonomy
- Simplification
- Structuring a safe environment
- Reminding a person often or offering multiple cues
- Repetition of routine – Routine, Routine, Routine . . . Same schedule, same caregivers, same daily routine
- Guidance & demonstration
- Reinforcement of good behaviors
- Stimulation to keep the person engaged
- Limited choices
- Avoiding open-ended questions
- Avoiding teaching new information i.e., attempting to make a person learn new things
- Minimizing demands on the person
- Minimizing anxiety
- Distraction
- Redirection
- Monitor for triggers of problematic behaviors
- Minimize distractions when a person is engaged in performing a task
- Minimize visual and auditory stimulation

(Zec & Burkett, 2008)

Problematic Behaviors & Suggestions for Management

Strategies to manage problematic behaviors exhibited by individuals suffering from dementia begin with acceptance of the person and the individual's present level of functioning. This includes valuing what the person is still able to do independently and not fixating on what a person is no longer able to do (Zec & Burkett, 2008). The key concept for caregivers to recognize is that a person's level of functioning will decline as the person's dementia progresses and, over time, the person will not be able to perform tasks as they once were able to do. Caregivers must be patient as well as develop strategies to deal with any issues as they arise – be flexible and go with the flow but create as much stability and routine as possible.

Agitation – Individuals in the moderate and later stages of dementia frequently become restless, anxious, or upset. To decrease agitation, listen to what the person is saying when expressing frustration to help identify the cause or trigger for the behavior; try to eliminate and/or decrease causes as much as possible. Potential causes for agitation include pain such as arthritis, constipation, pressure ulcers; discomfort such as being too hot, too cold, hungry, needing to urinate or have a bowel movement; frustration such as a person being upset when unable to remember how to perform a task or remember where a certain object was put; and over stimulation such as too much noise, lights, or an excessive number of people in the environment. It is also very important to examine the behavior of caregivers in response to a person's behaviors. Reassure an agitated person that caregivers are there to provide assistance and comfort. If an agitated person seems to be bored, then the person may need something to do – the caregiver may try to offer a distraction such as diverting the person's attention and providing them with an enjoyable activity.

Aggression – Some individuals suffering from dementia may exhibit aggressive behaviors such as shouting, cursing, cornering someone, throwing things, pushing, biting, or hitting. These problems can happen suddenly and sometimes without warning. Caregivers should attempt to identify any circumstances which may have triggered the aggression so that the cause can be eliminated or modified as soon as possible. Always try to react calmly, in a matter-of-fact manner and pay close attention to tone of voice and body language – both that of the caregiver and that of the person. Attempt to reassure the person in a soothing way and focus on the person's feelings. An upset person will often mirror the emotions of the caregiver and the manner in which the caregiver deals with an aggressive individual. And this can either improve the situation or escalate the problem. Monitor the person's environment and attempt to decrease as many distractions as possible such as loud noises, shadows, or movements. Be on the lookout for frustration which may escalate problems. Do not take combative behaviors personally – the person may be angry at a situation, a memory, or with their own abilities. Avoid teaching – instead offer encouragement. Assess the level of danger to the person and/or others to determine if the person's behaviors require management as well as how fast a caregiver must change the person's behavior. Use distraction and redirection of aggressive behaviors by changing the person's focus such as changing the subject or distracting a person with a different activity.

Repetition – Some individuals with dementia have repetitious behaviors such as repeating a word, question, or action over and over again for example saying "When will my daughter be here?" repeatedly. This type of behavior may be harmless but can be annoying for caregivers. Repetitive behaviors can be a sign of insecurity. Some individuals suffering from dementia may be seeking comfort and looking for something or someone who is familiar or attempting to create a situation in which they have some degree of control. To manage repetitive behaviors, attempt to identify a specific cause for the repetitive actions. Also investigate the emotions behind the behaviors, for example if the person appears distressed, angry, or depressed. Respond in a calm, patient manner and try turning the behavior into an activity that makes the person feel useful. For example, if the person is constantly fidgeting with her hands, try giving her washcloths to fold or a drawer to clean. If the person repeatedly asks questions – answer the person even if this happens several times a day. Consider using memory aides as reminders such as clocks, notes, calendars, and photographs. Engage the person in another activity to distract their attention.

Always stay calm and be patient. Provide a structured, repetitive routine. If not harmful, accept some behaviors, such as wandering, if the person is not trying to wander off and does not wander to the point of exhaustion.

Hallucinations – Visual hallucinations are seeing people or objects that are not real. Auditory hallucinations are hearing sounds or voices that are not real. Other hallucinations which are less common involve taste, smell, and touch – thinking someone or something is touching the person. Because hallucinations are real to the person, do not attempt to tell the person the hallucination is not real. Rather attempt to identify the person's feelings, reassure them you want to help, and redirect the person's attention to another activity. Also consider whether the hallucination is causing the person distress or if it is pleasant, such as seeing a loved one with whom they enjoy talking. If the hallucination is not disturbing, it may be more beneficial to agree with the person and not correct the person's belief. Consider asking for specifics about the hallucination to validate that you believe the person. Then repeat what the person is telling you about the hallucination so the person knows you are really listening.

Suspicion – A person with dementia may have difficulty accurately interpreting situations due to memory loss and disorientation. Suspicion is common – even the people close to the person may be targets of suspicion for a confused individual. This can include family members or caregivers. For example a confused person might accuse a caregiver of theft, infidelity, or other offenses. When suspicious behaviors occur, caregivers should not take the accusations personally. Remember these behaviors are caused by a disease that is affecting the person's personality and emotions. Imagine what it would be like to continuously wake up in a strange room, where you do not know anyone. They tell you when to eat and what to eat, when to bath, and what you can do as well as where you can go. You might think your possessions are being taken or hidden due to short-term memory impairment causing you to forget where you put your things. You have no control of your environment. Considering this viewpoint, caregivers may need to consider different strategies. Do not try to correct or argue with the suspicious person or convince them of your innocence when accused of things such as 'stealing' their belongings. Instead, offer assistance to the person, for example 'I see you are upset. What can I do to help?' One suggestion is to redirect a person's attention to another activity which has proven to be effective in these situations. Another suggestion is to have 'back-ups' or replacements of commonly misplaced items such as purses, hats, wallets, shoes, or shirts. This will allow the caregiver to 'locate' the missing object and to produce it when the person is searching for a favorite item.

Apathy – Lack of interest or motivation may not seem like a serious problem, but it is not healthy for someone suffering from dementia to simply sit and do nothing. Try to identify what may be triggering a person's apathy, such as being ignored or becoming overwhelmed with a decision or a task. Attempt to find out what may be reinforcing the behavior, such as being ignored or being scolded when unable to perform a certain task. Also determine if the person is being given too many choices or not being offered appropriate choices for pleasant activities. It is important to keep the person as active as possible to maintain physical and mental health as well as to decrease the incidence of depression. Try adapting activities to the person's level of functioning, both physically as well as cognitively, so the person can participate at a level that is comfortable and not overwhelming.

Confusion – Disorientation to person, place, and/or time. The person may know who they are but may not know where they are, what day it is, what month it is, or even the season or year. They may not recognize others and/or may mistake people they do not know for friends or relatives. An individual with dementia may develop Agnosia – an inability to recognize written words or an object, or Apraxia – confusion about how to use objects such as zippers or forks. Stay calm and provide simple, clear, positive

139

explanations and answers when the person asks for assistance. For example, if the person seems confused about the purpose of a spoon, tell the person, 'Here's a spoon, we use it for eating,' and show the person how to use it. Never be demeaning or use a scolding tone.

Sundowning – 'Sundowning' is the increase in confusion and increase in the occurrence of behaviors which are problematic in the late afternoon, early evening, and/or night-time hours – including agitation, aggression, and wandering. Sundowning is most commonly seen in individuals suffering from Alzheimer's disease but also occurs in individuals suffering from other dementias. Sundowning behaviors can occur as early as 2 to 3 p.m. but the most commonly reported time of occurrence is between 6 and 8 p.m. (Haggerly, 2002). There are several causes of sundowning including increased fatigue which can result in a decreased ability to tolerate stressful situations such as a noisy dinnertime or a bedtime routine; or increasing confusion, hallucinations, or delusions at night due to darkness and shadows. The best way to diminish sundowning behaviors is to establish a routine and engage the person involved in a non-demanding activity during the time the sundowning behaviors usually occur. For example, make late afternoons and evenings as simple and non-demanding as possible. Have the person fold washcloths in the afternoon – a repetitive, constructive activity. It is beneficial to reduce distractions and unscheduled activities at the times when these troubling behaviors usually escalate. Try to schedule routine activities in the morning when the person is more rested or when activities could be done at a different time of the day such as bathing. In the evening, keep rooms well-lit until bedtime to diminish shadows and hallucinations.

Wandering – Walking or propelling oneself in what appears to be a non-directional manner. This type of activity may be goal-directed but only the confused person knows the purpose. They may also have delusions and think they are going 'home' or to go pick up their children from school. Or this may be a non-goal directed type of wandering, for example the person wanders aimlessly up and down a hallway or from room to room. Wandering is not a bad activity unless it seems to upset the person, the person wanders to the point of exhaustion, the person will not eat, the person falls or injures him/herself, or the person wanders and becomes lost. Wandering can be a form of exercise as long as the person has a safe and structured environment. If the person is having problems due to wandering, ways to reduce the problem can include making sure the person has plenty of supervised activity to channel energies. Consider redirecting or diverting the person's attention to another activity. Or offer the person some form of distraction to divert their attention such as singing or painting (Hill, 2008).

Managing Wandering Behaviors when the
Person needs to be Re-Directed

- Approach a wanderer where you are seen – either from the side or front so not to startle the person
- Walk with the person, in the same direction the person was going initially or provide direction while walking with the person
- Guide the person in the direction you wish them to go, slowly turning so no sudden change in direction is apparent or make a circle to direct the person back to where you want the person to go
  - Abruptly reversing the direction (or turning the person around 90 degrees) may cause the person to become agitated
- Talk while walking with the person to offer distraction
- Take the person's hand, rather than grabbing the arm, to guide the person in the desired direction
- Reassure the person in a normal tone of voice
- Do not attempt to reorient the person who is agitated and intent on going somewhere or doing something
  - If person is disorientated – this could cause the person to become more agitated when told he/she is wrong about day, time, or place

---

Safety for Wanderers

Safety is one of the major concerns for caregivers of confused individuals who attempt to wander off and become lost or wander to places that could be potentially dangerous. If an individual tends to wander, it is optimal to create a safe and secure environment while allowing the person to maintain as much independence as possible – essentially allow the person to wander in an environment that has boundaries. Doors that are secure may help deter a wandering individual if there is a mechanism to prevent the person from accessing places they should not go – for example toddler covers for door-handles which prevent a person from opening a door or an electronic bracelet or anklet which causes a door to lock when the confused person attempts to exit. But there are times when a caregiver may have trouble locating a wandering person who has succeeded in going where they wish to go. It is essential to be prepared and have a plan of action in place.

If a Wanderer becomes lost: Develop a Plan of Action

- If the person wanders outside – be familiar with places to look or a trail the person usually follows
- Set time limit to call for help or to call 911 for help (call authorities for assistance to locate the person)
- Keep up-to-date photographs of the person
- Make sure to note what color clothing the person is wearing on a daily basis
- Make sure the person wears an identification bracelet or necklace which cannot be removed
- See the Safe Return program for ideas from the Alzheimer's Association

Managing Behaviors
Redirection

Redirecting and diverting an individuals' attention away from whatever the person is upset about or the stressful event to something that is more pleasant. For example, when a person insists 'I need to get to the kids from school,' offer to the person, 'Okay, but how about we see what's for dinner first since we have a few more minutes until the kids are out of school.' Obviously, this technique and its usefulness will depend upon what seems sensible in a given situation. Be creative and experiment to see what works and what doesn't with an individual. When redirection does not seem to be working, try asking pointed questions to get to the bottom of any unexplained behavior. It will make it easier to redirect if you understand what the person is thinking or why they are upset (Gilbert Guide 2009).

Validation Therapy

Validation therapy, first conceived by Naomi Feil, combines bluntly explaining reality with simply allowing individuals suffering from dementia to believe what they want to believe. Validation therapy integrates redirection techniques – moving an individual's attention from one thing to another and also validates an understanding of the person's feelings and emotions. Validation therapy is based on the idea that a person suffering from dementia may be sorting through past memories and past issues but living them out in the present. Some may even retreat to the past significantly, to restore a feeling of balance and control, especially if their present memory is failing. Allowing these individuals to live in their moments allows them some measure of control, which will aid in self-worth and will reduce the occurrence of negative behaviors (Gilbert Guide, 2009). Try to understand **why** the person is behaving a certain way, such as what may be the trigger or underlying concern. Then attempt to figure out how to address the issue. For example, if the person is hoarding or hiding items, ask what they are fearful of losing.

Give the person a "safe box" that can be used to store items that they are obsessed about. Do not attempt to make sense of a behavior, accept the behavior and the person. A person may seem lost or unable to complete a task and become frustrated – remember that the person's emotions are still valid and attempt to diminish frustrations by agreeing with the person's emotions. In fact, a distressing or anxious behavior can be amplified when the person is not accepted or not understood. Accept that a person's emotions have more validity than the logic that leads to the person becoming frustrated. Ask specific questions about how certain actions or situations make the person feel. After receiving an explanation of those feelings, validate feelings with phrases that show acceptance and support, such as, 'I'd be upset too, if that happened to me,' or 'I understand why you feel that way.' If a confused and agitated person wishes to leave, allow the person a graceful exit and be mindful of their ego! (Gilbert's Guide, 2009)

Supportive Measures to Diminish Problematic Behaviors

Individuals who are suffering from a diagnosis of dementia usually function better in familiar surroundings and in an established routine. Problematic behaviors occur less often when the person is within a structured and safe environment. Generally, the person's environment should be stable as well as include some stimulation such as an exercise program, stimulation from conversations, radio, or television. A person's environment should help with orientation of the person. For example, place the person near a window to enable differentiation of day and night or decorations for reminder of holidays.

Structure and routine will assist in orienting a confused person and give the person a sense of stability and security. When there are changes in routines, environment, or caregivers, simple and direct explanations should be given. Before every interaction, a confused person should be told what is going to happen, such as a bath or a meal. Taking time to explain can help prevent aggressive or combative behaviors. Following a daily routine for tasks can help a person suffering from dementia be able to remember to some degree. Establish a routine for bathing, eating, and sleeping (Merck, 2010).

Activities should be scheduled on a regular basis to help people suffering from dementia have a better quality of life, feel independent and needed and help relieve depression. Activities can be related to a person's interests prior to being diagnosed with dementia, should be enjoyable, and also provide stimulation but not be too challenging, which can cause frustration and aggression. Physical activity can relieve stress, expend a person's energy, and help prevent sleep problems and disruptive behaviors. Staying active also helps improve balance, which may help prevent falls and helps maintain (or improve) a person's overall health.

Engaging a person suffering from dementia in activities will assist in keeping the person more alert and possibly lead to the person having a better disposition. For example, a person should be stimulated with mental activities such as hobbies, interesting current events, and reading to the person about past events or reading old newspapers. Activities should not be demanding and may need to be broken down into small parts or simplified as a person's dementia worsens. A person with dementia should not be isolated, but excessive stimulation should also be avoided. Interaction with familiar people and socialization is encouraged. Activities should be incorporated into a simplified daily routine, expectations should be realistic, and structure should be predictable to maintain the person's dignity and self-esteem.

Environment

Keeping the environment simple and non-demanding with as few changes as possible has been shown to diminish behavioral problems in individuals suffering from dementia. A person's environment is the key to making their world as stress-free as possible.

Modifying Environment

Colors

- To draw a person's attention to something or somewhere – Use bright primary colors such as stark white, black, yellow, orange, and red
- For a calming effect – Use soothing colors (pastels) such as peach, pink, beige, ivory, light blues, greens, and lavender
- To assist in the person's ability to see objects more clearly, for example countertops, doorway to the bathroom, food from the plate – Use high contrast in colors such as red doorways with pastel walls, red plates on white tablecloths, or the plate a different color than the food
- To 'hide' things – Use similar colors such as doors the person should not use, attempt to make the color of the door and door-handle the same color as the wall
- Avoid use of busy patterns which can appear as movement to a person with depth perception issues (this problem is common in individuals with a diagnosis of dementia) such as in furniture, wallpaper, and flooring because this can have a negative impact on a person's balance and potentially cause falls
- Avoid shiny flooring or windows which may cause glare because these issues can prevent a person from seeing obstacles in their path. Consider use of diffuse lighting and covering windows with blinds, shades, or drapes

Simplistic

- Maintain a clutter-free environment because too many distractions or too many trinkets can be confusing and upsetting for confused individuals
- Clear the walking paths, especially to the bathroom and kitchen, of furniture which can cause falls

Orienting the Person to the Environment

- Use labels, pictures, and numbers to help individuals know where they are or what an object is
- Leave notes to remind individuals of things they need to do such as brush teeth, eat lunch, or change clothes

Safety
- Fall prevention
  - Area rugs or throw rugs can move when stepped upon and cause falls – use double sided tape on the backs of loose rugs
  - Use of socks increases a person's risk for slipping and falling – use socks with grippers on the bottom
  - Caution: poorly fitting shoes can cause falls. In addition, pets under the person's feet can also lead to falls.
- Decrease auditory stimulation
  - Use carpet which absorbs noise and prevents falls
  - Limit distractions and control noise levels
- Decrease visual stimulation which causes hallucinations or delusions
  - Avoid lighting which casts shadows, to diminish hallucinations
  - Use natural light and focus it directly on the areas where needed as much as possible
- Furniture – Use non-absorbent material to cover furniture or buy a comfortable recliner; Use primary colors and avoid busy patterns.
- Limit the use of certain appliances – electric razors, or hairdryers in the bathroom to reduce the risks of electrical shock
- Remove harmful objects which the person cannot use safely – cleaning solutions, knives, razors, power tools, or guns
- Be aware of plants which can be toxic if ingested
- Place medications where the person cannot get to them, to prevent overdosing

Safety Devices
- Place twist-bolt locks or child locks on doors to the exterior for wanderers and place the device either too high or too low so the person is unable to reach it and open the lock
- If using deadbolt locks – Keep an extra set of keys near the door for easy accessibility but out of sight for the person to use
- Remove locks from bathrooms or bedrooms so the person cannot get locked inside
- Childproof locks or door – knobs can assist in limiting access to the outside or to areas which contain harmful objects such as knives, equipment, cleaning supplies, or poisonous products
- Child gates can prevent a confused person from falling down stairs or entering rooms which are off-limits

Be Creative

- Use memory aids such as reminder notes, calendars, labels, or photographs
- Place large black rugs in front of doorways you do not wish a person to cross
  - Individuals with dementia have a problem with depth perception making rugs appears as holes and many individuals suffering from dementia may avoid walking over a dark rug
- Make doorknobs the same color as the door or cover the door with a picture so it blends into the wall
- Paint the door-frame a bright color different from the door's color for doors you wish the person to use, such as a bathroom
- If a person frequently hides an object and then thinks someone has stolen it, a person is always looking for a certain object, or a person wishes to wear the same shirt every day – Have multiples of the item to give the person when they become obsessed over the item

Bathing

- Have all necessary items for bath
- Have a warm environment
- Protect the person's privacy and dignity
- Allow the person to do as much of the bath as they can with minimal assistance
- If the person requires assistance- Remember Routine: Same caregiver and start with the same side of the body each time and work across
- If the person is resistant to a bath-decide if it is necessary-consider allowing the person to refuse a bath or put this task off until later
- If the bath is necessary and the person is resistant-consider creativity-offer a pedicure or a foot soak and then work your way to other body parts
- Distraction during the bathing process-talk or sing to the person to divert their attention
- Plan time of day and days of the week to bath-avoid 'sundowning' times

Caregivers who must manage problematic behaviors in confused individuals must be creative in developing strategies to prevent problems, diminish problems, and calm an agitated individual. Structuring the environment is essential and being knowledgeable of an array of maneuvers when one technique does not work will assist in decreasing the occurrence of problematic behaviors as well as diminish the problems when they do occur. Many times, approaches a caregiver takes can either make the situation better or cause it to become worse.

Non-pharmacologic Approaches to Management of Agitation/Aggression in Dementia

Techniques	Examples
Behavioral techniques	Validation therapy, Distraction, Operant conditioning, Limit setting, Providing limited choice, Differential reinforcement
Environmental modification	Structured Feeding assistance, Physical surroundings, Avoiding sensory overload
Group programs	Music, Exercise, Relaxation, Social skills training, Structured activities program
Light	Reduced intensity of lighting, Evening bright light pulses for individuals who frequently exhibit sundowning behaviors
Sound	Nature sounds, Soothing music
Touch	"Therapeutic touch"
Consistency in daily routine	Activities, Familiar possessions and clothing, Consistency in caregivers
Use of family members	Feeding, Environment
Communication	Improve caregivers' verbal and nonverbal communication skills to enhance resident's feelings of trust and safety

(Guay & Lott, 2010)

Managing Problematic Behaviors

When problematic behaviors occur, caregivers can take two approaches: Reactive – reacting to a behavior once a behavior occurs and/or Proactive – attempting to prevent a behavior from occurring or escalating.

Reactive strategies

- Redirection: distracting a confused individual and focusing attention on another activity or changing the topic of conversation. When having a person make a decision or choice, do not provide open-ended choices; limit the person to choosing between 2 or 3 options, but no more than 3. This will help prevent overwhelming the person and making the person freeze and thus make no decision. In offering a choice, make sure to pause to allow the person time to process the information and give a response.
  - Poor – What would you like to wear today?
  - Better – Would you like to wear the red shirt or the blue shirt?
- When a person seems upset, agitated, frustrated, or sad – Attempt to discover the cause of the problem or the reason for the belief or behavior
- Discover ways to find out what the person is trying to express or communicate by the behavior
- Crisis management – Utilize any and all strategies that work to calm an agitated person and prevent injury

Proactive strategies to prevent problems

- Create a stable routine and a structured environment. Or change an environment which is causing agitation or problematic behaviors to occur. Increase opportunities for access to a variety of activities but maintain a routine. Balance cognitively and physically demanding activities with periods of rest. Provide a predictable environment in order to reduce the level of cognitive demands on the person. Try to provide a consistent routine for waking, eating, toileting, grooming, and bathing. Make the home environment safe and free of objects that could be harmful. Be cautious in changing/moving furniture which changes the person's living space.

- Teach a simple way of performing a skill. These can include general skill development, useful communication strategies, and coping skills. Find activities which the person can do when feeling angry or anxious

- Individualize behavioral support plans. Reinforce specific desirable behaviors and attempt to ignore specific undesirable ones, unless they are dangerous. The main priority is to keep both the person and the caregiver safe through a crisis plan which might involve removing sharp objects or weapons, escaping to a safe place and giving the person time to calm down. Avoid activities which are known to upset the person and increase engagement in other activities.

When problematic behaviors occur, consider using an assertive tone in your response but do so in a nonjudgmental, clear, and unambiguous manner. This will provide a person with feedback that the behavior is not appropriate and then say what is preferred of the individual instead. For example, 'John, you're standing too close when we are talking; I feel uncomfortable, could you please move back a step or two?' Next, re-direct the person by changing the topic of discussion or diverting the person's attention to another activity. If any subsequent behavior occurs, attempt to ignore it. Finally attempt to understand what the behavior is trying to communicate and look at ways to have the need met in more appropriate ways.

Managing Inappropriate Behaviors

- Do not confront an aggressive, agitated person or try to discuss the angry behavior
- Do not initiate physical contact during an angry outburst
- Do not take the aggression personally
- Provide a time-out way from you (safe exit)
- Distract with a pleasurable topic or activity
- Look for patterns of aggression

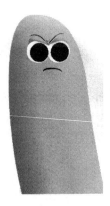

Physical Restraints

When confused individuals exhibit self-injurious behaviors or are potentially dangerous to others, non-pharmacological strategies should be implemented prior to resorting to physically restraining a person. There are some individuals who will require physical restraints, or the use of medications to calm potentially harmful behaviors which are not managed adequately with non-pharmacologic measures alone. The use of physical restraints includes arm and leg ties, Posey jackets, lap belts/sheets, mittens, bed rails, and restraining chairs. Restraints are not recommended for use on a long term basis and are considered inhumane, can constitute cruel and unusual punishment, and involve loss of autonomy (Guay & Lott, 2010).

There have been numerous medical issues surrounding the use of physical restraints due to the potential consequences of limb ischemia, asphyxiation, neuropathy, aspiration, bone resorption, decubiti, urinary retention, fecal impaction, enhanced agitation, and even death if improperly applied. There has been little evidence to indicate that physical restraints achieve the goals of protecting the restrained individual, protecting others, or preventing falls and may, in fact, result in further injuries. Restraints should be avoided through use of alternative techniques including environmental structuring, behavior modification, and caregiver education. This includes caregiver toleration of bothersome but benign behaviors such as sleep disturbances, wandering, and restlessness (Guay & Lott, 2010).

Restraints should only be used in emergency situations when an individual's behavior represents an immediate danger to him/herself or others and the use of restraints is considered the best alternative. Restraints should not be used for prevention of falls or control of agitation, especially on a daily basis and without consent. If restraints are necessary, the restraint should be padded and the individual should checked every 30-60 minutes, with removal of the restraint from each limb and assessment of basic needs of the person at least hourly. There should be an assessment for abrasions and pressure areas conducted every three to four hours (Guay & Lott, 2010).

Medication Management for Challenging Behaviors

In certain individuals who exhibit problematic behaviors, medications may be a last resort to management of the problems. There are no medications indicated or approved to treat the behavioral problems exhibited by individuals suffering from dementia. But medications are often used and may be necessary when the problematic behaviors become unmanageable, the individual is in danger of harming self or others, and the person's quality of life is extremely poor due to the behaviors. The maintenance medications have been discussed in the preceding chapters on the different dementias. The following table lists other medications commonly used to manage problematic behaviors in individual with dementia. NOTE: There are no medications approved by the FDA to treat or manage problematic behaviors in individuals with a diagnosis of dementia, including Alzheimer's disease dementia, but the following are the medications commonly prescribed and used in practice when caring for these problems. This discussion is necessary so caregivers are aware of the intent of their use, the proper geriatric dosing recommendations, the potential hazards, and proper oversight if a medication is used.

Medications Commonly Used to Manage Coexisting Behavioral Problems in Individuals Suffering from Dementia

Antipsychotic Medications: The first generation medications are frequently prescribed to help manage psychosis and agitation. This class includes haloperidol (Haldol), risperidone (Risperdal), olanzapine (Zyprexa), and quetiapine (Seroquel). Treatment of dementia-associated psychosis or agitation is intended to decrease psychotic symptoms such as paranoia, delusions, hallucinations, screaming, combativeness, spitting, self-mutilation, and/or violence. The goal is to increase comfort and safety of individuals, families, and caregivers as well as improve the person's quality of life. Attention should be given to monitor for adverse effects including dystonia (see below), falls, increased confusion, orthostatic hypotension (blood pressure falls when the person stands), or any other problems.*

The second generation antipsychotic medications include ziprasidone HCl (Geodon) and aripiprazole (Abilify). These medications can have the same problematic adverse effects listed for the first generation antipsychotic medications. In addition, with ziprasidone, attention should be given to monitor for a potentially life-threatening problem known as Q-on-T phenomenon – an abnormality of the heart's rhythm which can cause ventricular tachycardia and death – it is encouraged for any individual taking this medication to have an Electrocardiogram

(EKG) routinely done – prior to initiating the medication and at least every 3 months while on this medication.

All antipsychotic medications have the following potential complications: strokes, heart attack, worsening of cholesterol, development of or worsening of diabetes, falls, and orthostatic hypotension.

Monitoring: Laboratory values should be done periodically. The first year of therapy – every 3 months initially then every 6 to 12 months thereafter: Liver function, Kidney function, Cholesterol levels, and control of or development of diabetes (Hgb A1C).

Weaning off the medication: Only use an antipsychotic medication when absolutely necessary and consider weaning the person off the medication if possible. After initiating a medication, allow the person's behaviors to calm and then maintain the medication usage for 2 to 3 months. Then begin reducing the dose slowly and attempt to wean the person off the medication – diminish the medication by ½ the current dose for 2 to 4 weeks and then continue reduction until the person is no longer taking the medication. If the person's agitation and behaviors recur, consider increasing the medication dose back to the dose which managed the problem or prevented the problematic behaviors. Consider a second trial to wean a person off the medication. Re-attempt to wean the dose again after 3 months. If the behaviors are not tolerable when this medication is decreased or stopped, the person may have greater benefit from being maintained on the medication than having the medication stopped. But judicious monitoring for problems should be done.

Antidepressant medications: Depression is frequently associated with dementia and generally worsens the degree of cognitive and behavioral impairment. Antidepressants have been shown to improve quality of life and diminish problematic behaviors in individuals suffering from dementia.

Antidepressant medications (continued): There are many classes of antidepressant medications but Selective Serotonin reuptake Inhibitors (SSRIs) are a class of antidepressants which is the safest and most effective for use in older individuals with dementia. This class includes duloxetine (Cymbalta), escitalopram (Lexapro), paroxetine (Paxil), paroxetine CR (Paxil CR), fluoxetine (Prozac), sertraline (Zoloft), citalopram (Celexa), and venlafaxine XR (Effexor XR).

Antianxiety drugs: Many patients with dementia experience anxiety symptoms. Anxiolytic medications include benzodiazepines, which are considered a narcotic medication. Examples of this include alprazolam (Xanax), diazepam (Valium), lorazepam (Ativan), and clonazepam (Klonipin). They have been used for treating anxiety with anxious conditions that are not caused by dementia. They are often avoided in older adults with a diagnosis of dementia because these medications may increase agitation in certain persons or can be sedating. The shorter anxiolytics (Ativan or Xanax) are preferred if one of this class of medication is ultimately necessary and it is encouraged to only be used on an 'as needed basis' for anxiety and not scheduled to be given routinely. Caution should be exercised to monitor for falls or orthostatic hypotension. A non-narcotic alternative may be buspirone (Buspar) which can be used to manage mild-to-moderate anxiety.

(Kalapatapu & Schimming, 2009; eMedicine.Net, 2010)

Dystonia

Dystonia is a neurological movement disorder, in which sustained muscle contractions cause twisting and repetitive movements or abnormal postures. It can occur as an adverse effect caused by medications such as an antipsychotic medication. If a person starts exhibiting a dystonia – the clinician should consider if the medication should be continued. Dystonia is an abnormal movement problem which can occur after starting on an antipsychotic medication and may persist even after the medication is stopped. The benefits of continuing the medication should be weighed against the risks of this becoming a permanent problem. Consider discontinuing the medication if any of these problems develop.

Dystonia

Type	Location	Description
Cervical dystonia (spasmodic torticollis)	muscles of the neck	A person's head to rotates to one side, may pull down towards the chest or back, or the person may assume a combination of these postures
Blepharospasm	muscles around the eyes	Rapid blinking of the eyes or even forced closure of eyes causing effective blindness
Oculogyric crisis	muscles of eye and head	An extreme and sustained, usually upward deviation of the eyes, often with convergence causing diplopia (double vision); it is frequently associated with backwards and lateral flexion of the neck and either widely opened mouth or jaw clenching
Oromandibular dystonia	muscles of the jaw and muscles of tongue	Muscle spasms causing distortions of the mouth and tongue

Type	Location	Description
Spasmodic dysphonia/ Laryngeal dystonia	muscles of larynx	Spasms which cause the voice to sound broken or reduce it to a whisper
Focal hand dystonia (also known as musician's or writer's cramp) (Mayo Clinic, 2009; Wikipedia, 2010)	single muscle or small group of muscles in the hand	Involuntary muscle contractures which interfere with activities such as writing or playing a musical instrument. The condition is sometimes 'task-specific' meaning that it generally only occurs during certain activities. Focal hand dystonia is neurological in origin and is not due to normal fatigue. The loss of precise muscle control and continuous unintentional movement results in painful cramping and abnormal positioning that makes continued use of affected body parts impossible.

Chapter 6 References

Alzheimer's Society: Leading the fight against dementia. (2008). Retrieved 7-29-2008 from www.alzheimers.org.uk/site/ scripts/documents_info.php?documentID=159

eMedicine.Net (2010) Dementia-Medications. Retrieved April 9, 2010 from http://www.emedicinehealth.com/dementia_ medication_overview/page6_em.htm

Gilbert Guide (2009). How to Talk to an Elder with Dementia Using Validation Therapy, Redirection & Other Techniques. Retrieved May 26, 2010 from http://www.psgdc.org/GG_ article1.html

Hagerly, D. (2002). The safety program sunset for sundowning: this facility's staff came up with plans to attack the most hazardous part of many residents' day – 2002 Optima Award Winner – some elderly show increased activity around sundown. *Nursing Homes.*

Hill, C. (2010). Behavior Management: How to Manage the Challenging Behaviors of Alzheimer's Disease. *About.com Guide.* 2-28-2008. Retrieved April 7, 2010 from http:// alzheimers.about.com/od/caregiving/a/behaviors.htm

Kalapatapu, R. & Schimming, C. (2009). Update on neuropsychiatric symptoms of dementia: Antipsychotic use. *Geriatrics.* 64 (5). 10-18.

Mayo Clinic. (2009). Healthletter: Dystonia. 27(12). 6.

Merck Manual. (2010). Dementia. Retrieved March 25, 2010 from http://www.merck.com/mmhe/sec06/ch083/ch083c.html

Norrgard, C., & Matheis-Kraft, C. (2006). Difficult behaviors associated with Alzheimer's disease. *Senior Health Advisor.* Retrieved 7/28/2008 from www.fairview.org/ healthlibrary/content/print_sha_alzprobs_sha.htm

Russell, D., Barston, S., & White, M. (2007). Alzheimer's behavior management: learn to manage common behavior problems. Retrieved 7-29-2008 from www.helpguide.org/elder/

alzheimers_behavior_problems.htm

Wikipedia. (2010). Disinhibition. Retrieved April 7, 2010 from
http://en.wikipedia.org/wiki/Disinhibition

Wikipedia. (2010). Dystonia. Retrieved April 9, 2010 from http://
en.wikipedia.org/wiki/Dystonia

Zec, & Burkett, (2008). Non-pharmacological and pharmacological
treatment of the cognitive and behavioral symptoms of
Alzheimer's disease. NeuroRehabilitation Journal (23).
425-438.

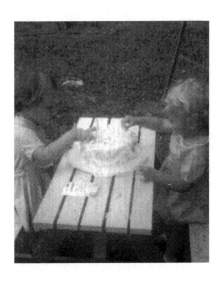

Chapter 7

Eating is the last activity of daily living lost by an individual suffering from dementia. There are many physical as well as psychiatric issues affecting an individual's ability to eat. This chapter will review of the complexity of the eating process and present strategies to enhance and improve the nutritional status of individuals with a diagnosis of dementia.

Introduction

Eating is essential for staying alive and being healthy. But eating, in our society, is more than just maintaining life and sustenance. It is something that is celebrated – people get together for holidays, birthdays, and special occasions. It is ritualistic – we have meals with 'the family' or with friends. And it is a source of enjoyment because people like to eat different foods and go to different places according to food preferences. Eating is one of the last functions of the activities of daily living to be lost by individuals with dementia. There are many reasons why confused individuals decrease their intake. Loss of memory and problems with judgment can cause many difficulties which may manifest themselves in all stages of a disease that causes dementia; the early problems can begin with:

- Problems with shopping – inability to decide what to buy or unable to make appropriate food selections
- Inability to cook – unable to understand how the stove works, how to prepare food – carry out a recipe, or how to recognize utensils
- Inability to eat – sometimes the damage to the brain may affect the person's ability to carry out the sequential steps of eating

Eating Problems in Elders with Dementia

     An individual suffering from dementia may have declining abilities which will have an effect on nutrition and hydration throughout the course of the person's illness. In the early stage of dementia, an individual may forget to eat, may become depressed and not want to eat, or may become distracted and leave the table without eating. As the disease progresses, the individual with dementia may be easily distracted and unable to sit long enough to eat. Yet, at this stage, a person may require an additional 600 calories per day because of wandering and motor restlessness or a person may be chair-bound and require fewer calories. In the late stage of a dementia, an individual may forget the sequence of steps to eating and may not have intact oral motor skills for chewing and swallowing, which can lead to malnourishment and begin a cascade of decline or cause a person to begin to 'waste away' (Curfman, 2005). Eating is a complex process – see the following discussion of the steps of eating.

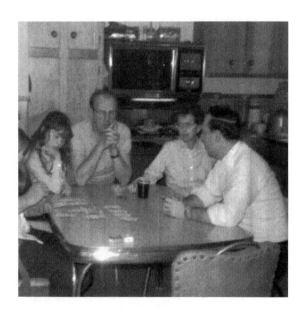

Steps of Eating

- **Oral preparatory phase**
  - prepare the food into a bite small enough to place in the mouth which can be chewed
- **Oral phase – chew the food and prepare the bolus of food to swallow**
  - food is placed in the mouth and chewed
  - food is mixed with saliva and reshaped by chewing it to a consistency which can be swallowed
- **Pharyngeal – swallowing**
  - breathing ceases momentarily as the bolus of food is moved through the pharynx
  - the nasopharynx is sealed with the elevation of the soft palate
  - the tongue pushes the bolus through the pharynx via sequential pressure waves
  - just milliseconds before the onset of the pharyngeal contraction, the hyoid & larynx move upward to close the laryngeal vestibule and airway entrance, thereby preventing aspiration
  - upper esophageal sphincter (UES) opens to allow the bolus to enter the esophagus
  - as the tail of the bolus passes the UES, the pharyngeal structures return to rest & breathing begins again
- **Esophageal**
  - the food bolus moves to the stomach through muscular action – peristalsis
    - » peristalsis is the product of the reciprocal relaxation & contraction of the circular and longitudinal muscles that make up the esophagus
  - Lastly – at rest, the esophagus relaxes and is a collapsed, closed tube with a sphincter at each end

Appetite

In many individuals suffering from dementia, there can be problems with their appetite center. Some of the different problems include: a) **Overeating or insatiable appetite** – consider offering 5 or 6 small meals per day; have low-calorie snacks available; distract the person with other activities such as walking or singing; and it may be necessary to lock up some foods; b) **Under-eating** – consider offering a glass of juice or wine to stimulate appetite; offer ice cream or eggnogs; increase exercise; try offering all or more of one food before offering the next to avoid change of taste and texture; have main meal coinciding with the time of the day when the person is at their best – usually the middle of the day; offer familiar or favorite foods; and c) **Sweet cravings** – consider offering milk shakes or eggnogs as an alternative; offer low calorie ice cream and high protein 'sweets', or sweets made with whole grains and vegetables (myDoc, 2010).

In some individuals, hunger sensations may no longer be interpreted by the damaged brain and a person is unaware of the necessity to eat. The person may forget they have already eaten and are always seeking food or forget to eat at all. And some medications, as well as concurrent medical problems a person can have, may cause potential side effects such as affecting appetite or causing nausea and/or indigestion.

Symptoms of Eating Problems in Individuals
Suffering from Dementia

- Extra effort to chew or swallow
- Eating very slowly
- Packing food in cheeks or holding food in mouth
- Swallowing several times for a single mouthful of food
- Shortness of breath during eating
- Coughing or choking while eating or drinking
- Drooling
- A wet-sounding voice after eating
- Hoarseness after meals
- Increased congestion in the chest after eating
- Repeated bouts of pneumonia

Determining the Problem Related to Eating & Nutrition

Individuals suffering from dementia can have a variety of problems related to eating and nutrition, and the key to treating the problem is determining the cause of the problem. Many individuals with dementia are easily distracted, some are unable to interpret the sensations of hunger and thirst, some forget they are eating or forget the steps of the eating process, and some have dysphagia – a mechanical problem with swallowing either due to nerve damage, muscle damage, or the brain's control of movement of the muscles of swallowing. Observation of a person's eating habits will provide many clues to the cause of the problem.

Distraction

Many individuals with dementia are easily distracted when eating, which can lead to malnutrition and other problems including aspiration. Imagine being in a busy restaurant with a group of friends, there is loud music playing close or you are sitting in a high traffic area with people walking by frequently. There is a lot of activity in the restaurant and the conversations around the table are loud. Ordering requires making a choice from a long list of options on the menu as well as keeping up with the conversations at the table. The waiter is hovering and you are feeling pressure to choose, to order. It may be challenging to concentrate on the conversations around the table while choosing from the menu, but you will manage to make a decision, order, and continue to converse with the people at the table despite everything else going on in the restaurant. For individuals with dementia, a noisy environment can be confusing: it can further increase difficulty in a person's ability to concentrate and focus. Some individuals with dementia cannot tolerate this type of environment and feel compelled to escape – some are able to do this and maneuver away. But others cannot and are trapped, possibly becoming overwhelmed by their surroundings. Being aware that individuals with dementia are overwhelmed when over-stimulated by their environment and understanding how these individuals may struggle to concentrate at mealtimes if there are distractions – will assist caregivers in developing an appropriate meal-time environment for these individuals. It is encouraged that a confused person's eating environment be calm and relaxed with minimal distractions, if possible (SCIE, 2010).

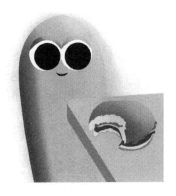

**Eating Environment can Hinder Eating for
Individuals with Dementia**

- Activity
- Noise
- Distractions (conversations, shows, music, people walking by)
- Lighting
- Seating (friendship, need for assistance to eat, etc)
- Choices of foods
- Differing diets at the same table

Individuals suffering from dementia may not feel relaxed and comfortable eating with other people or in an unfamiliar environment. Others may have difficulty eating food due to frequent spills or may just become paranoid. Any of these issues can only make feelings of embarrassment worse if sitting with others. As a result, the person may leave food uneaten even when hungry. Allow a person to sit and eat in a place where they feel comfortable, either at a table or perhaps sitting with a tray on their lap in a comfortable chair. But socialization is encouraged to keep a person interacting with others as well as for safety reasons – to prevent a person from choking and no-one being aware of the problem if the person was eating alone (SCIE, 2010).

Vision

There are many changes to a person's vision associated with normal aging which affect eating, including a decreased ability to see objects that are close – a majority of older individuals develop farsightedness or presbyopia; for example, the person sees something in front of them but is unaware it is food because they cannot see it clearly. Many older individuals have difficulty seeing objects of similar color, for example light-colored mashed potatoes disappear on a white plate. Also affected by aging is depth perception and this is more pronounced in individuals with Alzheimer's disease; for example, the person cannot estimate how much food is on their plate or not realize that they have not eaten enough food. Untreated vision problems in older age are also associated with an increased risk of decline in cognitive function and hastening the progression of certain dementias including Alzheimer's disease (Bankhead, 2010).

Normal Aging Changes to Vision

- **Depth perception**: The cornea, which refracts light, becomes flatter, less smooth, and thicker making older eyes more susceptible to astigmatism.
- **Decreased ability to differentiate colors**: There is a yellowing of the lens causing some reduction of the eye's ability to discriminate blues, greens, and violets; yellows, oranges, and reds are seen more clearly.
- **Ptosis**: Eyelids may droop as elasticity diminishes leading to occlusion of the visual field.
- **Dry Eyes**: Decrease in orbicular muscle strength causes an eyelid to stay open slightly, leading to corneal dryness which can cause blurry vision.
- **Presbyopia**: After 40 years of life, the eye losses the ability to accommodate to close objects and this problem continues to worsen or progress throughout a person's life. This makes it difficult for a person to identify what food is on their plate.
- **Decreased Peripheral Vision**: Peripheral vision decreases making a person's visual field less as well as causing difficulty in seeing objects or people approaching which are not directly in front of the person or can make items disappear such as the person seeing only the items in the center of the plate and foods on the edges may not be seen.
- **Slower Pupil Accommodation**: Pupil size is smaller creating a slower constriction in the presence of bright light. There is a slowing of the pupil's dilation in dark settings and a slowing in the ability to accommodate to changes in light. Glare occurs

often in sunlight as well as light reflecting off shiny objects. Older eyes need three times more light, making night vision impaired for older adults.

- **Glaucoma**: The anterior chamber of the eye decreases as the thickness of the lens increases. In some older individuals, there is an increase in the density of collagen fibers leading to inefficient resorption of intraocular fluids and glaucoma.

- **Cataracts**: Lens opacities can develop after the age of 50 causing a cloudiness in vision which can progress to obscure vision completely as well as cause everything to appear blurred.

- **Opacities** can develop and can be seen as spots or clusters of dots in the visual field which are coalesced vitreous that have broken off the periphery or central part of the retina. These are largely harmless although they can be annoying and potentially cause visual hallucinations and paranoia.

How Alzheimer's Disease Affects Vision More Markedly in Older Adults

Older Adults suffering from Alzheimer's disease:
- Have a decreased ability to perceive color contrasts
- Have more markedly impaired depth perception – trouble identifying foods and quantity of foods
  - » objects close together or on top of each other are also similar in color or value which causes foods to disappear from the individual's vision
- Visualize colors as lightness or darkness, appearing more on a gray scale than a color scale
- Have more tunnel vision, making it harder to see close to the edges of objects
- Short term memory impairment can affect remembering food has not been eaten, for example foods which may drop off the plate may be forgotten since the person no longer sees the food – the person believes they have eaten the food

Hearing & Auditory Distractions

A noisy environment may make eating difficult for individuals with dementia who are easily distracted. Adding to this problem is hearing deficits. Many individuals have some degree of hearing loss, making certain sounds and consonants difficult to hear – when trying to listen to conversations in their surroundings, they may only hear bits and pieces of words and conversations due to loss of certain sounds which can lead to delusions and paranoia in some confused individuals.

Auditory Distractions that Affect Eating for Individuals with Dementia

- Some individuals find it hard to keep the conversations in the same room
- Hearing deficits can cause fragmentation of conversations the person hears, making the person paranoid and suspicious
- Background noises cause distractions or frighten a person who does not understand what the sound is
  - » ice machines
  - » metallic clanging of silverware
  - » announcements on the public-address system
  - » a radio or boom box playing "dinner" music
- Many individuals with dementia find it hard to cope with the stimulation associated with group dining

Changes to Taste & Smell in Normal Aging

A person's sense of taste and smell diminish as they age. These two senses interact closely, helping an individual taste and appreciate food. People have approximately 9,000 taste buds, which are primarily responsible for sensing as well as differentiating sweet, salty, sour, and bitter tastes. The number of taste buds decreases as individuals age, beginning at about age 40 to 50 in women and at 50 to 60 in men – the remaining taste buds also begin to atrophy or be lost. A person's ability to taste certain foods changes over time, making food preferences change. The sense of smell enhances a person's ability to taste foods and, as the sense of smell diminishes with normal aging, the ability to taste foods will also change.

The sense of smell begins at nerve receptors high in the membranes of the nose and with normal wear and tear, these receptors can become dislodged and diminish a person's ability to smell. Although most older individuals have a decline in their sense of smell with normal aging, it has been found that this loss is more pronounced in individuals suffering from Alzheimer's disease. Smell (and to a lesser extent, taste) play a role in both safety and enjoyment. A delicious meal or pleasant aroma can improve social interaction and enjoyment of life. But certain smells can alert a person that something is not safe to eat or something is not an edible object.

The ability to taste is usually lost in a specific pattern. Usually, salty and sweet tastes are lost first, with bitter and sour tastes lasting slightly longer. Many individuals with dementia will attempt to eat very salty foods and eat sweets frequently to satisfy their need for these tastes. Additionally, a person's mouth produces less saliva with aging which can cause a dry mouth, contributing to difficulty in swallowing. It also makes digestion slightly less efficient and can increase dental problems because with an adequate amount of saliva-food particles are washed off teeth – without removal of food particles, there is an increased development of caries which can lead to tooth breakage, tooth loss, gingivitis, and illness (MedLine Plus, 2010).

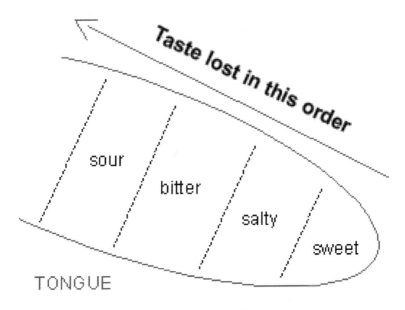

Figure 12: Changes in Taste

Dysphagia

Dysphagia is chewing and/or swallowing problems, which can be life threatening for older individuals. The muscles of the mouth and throat may no longer be working properly, allowing bits of food and liquid to be aspirated or inhaled into the lungs, which can lead to respiratory infections, pneumonia and, potentially, death. Other factors contributing to dysphasia include a person's level of consciousness (how alert a person is), medications, distractions and eating patterns.

When a person aspirates either food or fluids, the passages of the lungs become blocked; the person may begin to choke or may not – which is known as 'silent aspiration'. For frail, elderly individuals, a choking fit can be fatal. Aspiration of food and fluid into the lungs can cause aspiration pneumonia, which is a potentially deadly problem in individuals with dementia and is more prevalent

172

in individuals who are in the final stage of dementia. Repeated bouts of aspiration pneumonia will weaken a person's system and may eventually cause death (How to care, 2010).

Chewing Problems

Chewing problems in individuals suffering from dementia may be related to cognition problems or poor dental health including missing teeth or poorly fitting dentures. Properly fitted dentures, proper oral hygiene before and after meals, and regular dental visits may help minimize some of these problems.

Signs of Chewing and Swallowing Problems

- Extra effort chewing or swallowing
- Eating very slowly
- Packing food into the cheeks
- Swallowing several times for a single mouthful of food
- Shortness of breath during eating
- Coughing or choking while eating or drinking
- Drooling
- Fluid leaking from the nose after swallowing
- A wet-sounding voice after eating
- Increased congestion in the chest after eating
- Repeated bouts of pneumonia

If an individual is suspected of having problems with either silent aspiration or overt aspiration (coughing or choking when drinking and/or eating) and has repeated bouts of respiratory infections or other signs of aspiration, attempt to identify what could be causing the problem:

- What was the person doing when the coughing/choking occurred such as talking, laughing, walking
- What type of food or fluid was he/she eating when the coughing or choking occurred, such as thin liquids, breads, hard to chew meats

- If the person wears dentures, were they in at the time of the choking episode? Do the dentures fit properly?

(How to Care, 2010)

Getting Help

If there are concerns about a person's eating or drinking abilities, there are some key healthcare professionals who can offer advice and guidance:

- Dietitians – provide advice on issues such as poor appetite, weight loss or weight gain, food enrichment and vitamin and food supplements
- Speech and language therapists – give advice and guidance on swallowing difficulties. It is important that changes to the texture of food are only made as necessary and with their professional advice
- Occupational therapists – advice on adaptive eating aids, such as cutlery, cups and plate mats, that help to maintain independent eating

---

(Alzheimer's Association, 2010)

Assessing Eating Problems

When an individual suffering from dementia is having problems eating and potentially problems with dysphagia (difficulty swallowing), an initial assessment is done to identify the nature of the dysphagia, identify any contributing factors, differentiate physiologic impairment and cognitive dysfunction factors, identify ways to improve safety, and identify the person's ability to benefit from skilled intervention. Assessment begins with identification of the problem and the effects it has on a person. The first step is to observe a person's eating abilities and then interview the person to assist in identifying the problem. It is also helpful to obtain information from any person who has observed any eating problem or episodes of dysphagia. After an assessment of a person's abilities, it is necessary to examine many other factors including: sensory function, head and neck positioning, oral motor skills, and swallowing skills such as patterns of mastication, salivation, and laryngeal elevation (Curfman, 2005).

Fortunately, the effect of a progressive dementia on swallowing functioning can be fairly predictable. An assessment of the person's cognitive abilities is imperative and will include assessment of recent recall or ability to follow instructions although this may be limited because of memory impairment, dementia, or other language deficits. Therefore, the following information should be sought:

---

* all diagnoses, including the type of dementia
* current weight as well as any recent weight changes
  o prefer weights over the last 6 months to assess weight fluctuations or for a trend of continued weight loss
* current diet as well as any recent changes in diet
* current eating habits, including food types and amounts consumed at scheduled & unscheduled times
* self-feeding skills throughout the course of each meal and throughout the day
* eating and chewing difficulties
* signs/symptoms of hoarseness or wet-sounding voice after meals, runny nose after meals, congestion, coughing, choking with drinking or taking medications, fever, and lethargy
* Radiological test results (chest x-ray and modified barium swallow)
* history of respiratory infections and/or pneumonia

Observation is the initial step in assessing an eating problem and begins with observing the person at mealtime to see if the problem can be identified. During an individual interview with the person having eating difficulties, there are two key questions:

(1) What are the problems with eating, drinking, and swallowing? And (2) Why does the person think he/she is having a problem with swallowing? Valuable information about a person's perception of the problem, cognitive status, and ability to attend to and follow directions as well as learn new information will influence the nature of the treatment plan. Many individuals with dementia who have dysphagia, also have a neurologic impairment which will make the person unable to understand questions or unable to follow instructions and may hinder participation in the interview process. Expressive aphasia is an inability to verbalize what a person is thinking and Receptive aphasia is an inability to understand what they are being told. Other issues which can cause problems include cognitive dysfunction which is an inability to understand terms being used in the questioning process or an inability to comprehend what is being asked. If these issues are hindering the initial assessment of the problem, the necessary information may be obtained from people who have observed the problem and are familiar with the individual and then direct observation can be conducted to identify the basic problem(s).

Sensory function. It is important to determine whether the person has problems with sensory pathways. The following six anatomic sites are assessed to determine if a sensory deficit is causing problems with eating. Assessment is conducted in the following order:

---

* tongue (anterior two-thirds)
* tongue (posterior one-third)
* hard palate
* soft palate
* posterior pharyngeal wall
* laryngeal region

(Curfman, 2005)

Some sensory problems that may contribute to a decrease in a person's intake can be an altered or absent perception of taste;

diminished safety mechanism for sensing hot food, with potential/ actual injuries of the mouth; and/or profound sensory loss in the later stages of the dementia that hinder a person's ability to chew and swallow.

Head and neck positioning. Assessment of the position a person maintains when eating – both the body position as well as the position of the person's head, should be done if an individual is able to sit when instructed to do so. A person may require assistance in positioning and caregivers should be assessed in how they position an individual for mealtimes. Three common head/neck positions that occur in the later stages of dementia include:

1. chronic head/neck flexion (head bent forward)
2. variable head/neck flexion/extension caused by a lack of positioning management (inability to hold head upright)
3. chronic head/neck hyperextension (head positioned backward)

The main goal in the late stage of dementia is to improve the individual's ability to eat through the use of adaptive equipment or assistive devices. It is encouraged to attempt to maintain an individual in an upright position while eating: sitting upright with the head flexed at a 90 degree angle to simulate as close to the way a person has eaten most of their lives.

Oral motor skills. Visual assessment of an individual's eating ability consists of watching and assessing motion and movement, strength, and coordination of individual oral structures (lips, tongue – anterior, middle, and posterior, and soft palate); and assessing the functional movement patterns required for the oral stage of swallowing, including manipulation of food during chewing, cohesive food bolus formation, anterior-to-posterior transit of cohesive food bolus, and later stage of swallowing – the transfer or dropping of food bolus into pharynx.

Pattern of mastication. Assessment of mastication involves assessing the muscles associated with chewing and the pattern of chewing/swallowing. The function of the oral musculature will determine the pattern of mastication, which will deteriorate in a predictable fashion with the progression of an individual's dementia. The progressive deterioration in the mastication patterns below reflects a transition from higher level reflex integration to lower level reflex integration during the course of a person's dementia:

---

* rotary chew pattern
* lateral chew/chomping pattern and jaw – jaw jerk reflex
* suck – swallow pattern
* absent oral motor function for chewing

(Curfman, 2005)

Salivation. Assessment of salivary function includes inspecting the oral mucosa visually to determine adequacy of salivary flow, review of medications, and review of medical history. There are many common medications that can reduce salivation including the following classes of medications: anticholinergic agents, antidepressants, and antipsychotic drugs. If salivary flow is adequate, the oral cavity (mouth) will appear moist; if hyposalivation (low salivary production), the oral cavity will become dry. Symptoms of dry mouth or xerostomia include mouth pain; difficulty chewing; difficulty swallowing; weight loss; mouth infections; tooth decay; a dry, cracked tongue; bleeding gums; cracked corners of the mouth; badly fitting dentures; and dryness in the eyes, nose, skin, and throat. If a person appears to have a dry mouth or complains about a dry mouth, the person should be assessed for other signs/symptoms of dehydration, including dry mucous membranes; loss of skin turgor; intense thirst; flushed skin; oliguria (which is decreased urine output); concentrated urine which appears as dark yellow or brown urine; and/or possible elevated temperature (Curfman, 2005).

Analyzing volitional swallows and laryngeal elevation. Once swallowing is initiated, it should occur briskly. The observer should assess if elevation of the larynx occurs during dry and/or bolus swallows. The components of laryngeal elevation would include the speed of laryngeal elevation, the movement of the structures involved, and the integrity of their movement.

Dysphagia of Dementia

The following are secondary conditions related to the primary diagnosis of dementia:

---

* absent oral motor pattern for chewing
* poor sensory awareness
* negative reaction to food textures and consistencies
* suck – sawllow mastication pattern
* significant irreversible pharyngeal dysphagia
* reduced intake by mouth secondary to behavioral issues

Treatment in Individuals with Dementia and Dysphagia

There are ways to improve dysphagia in individuals with dementia. Treatment can be divided into direct treatment, preferably by a trained professional – usually a speech therapist who works directly with a person, teaching him/her strategies to improve the problem: sensory stimulation, diet modification, muscle strengthening, and caregiver training in feeding assistance. And indirect treatment, preferably by a trained professional, usually a speech therapist who sets up an individualized plan of care which incorporates environmental modifications, adaptive equipment/ assistive devices, and safety strategies to be used by a designated caregiver: addition of sweetener to food items (if only sweet taste receptors remain); use of alternative nutritional systems, such as enteral feeding (tube feeding a person); and/or oral care/sensory stimulation provided by caregiver (Curfman, 2005).

179

Treatment suggestions may include:

* sensory stimulation
    » increasing texture variation (dry crackers or crisp cookies)
    » increasing mouth sensation
    » facilitating mastication (chewing) pattern
* diet management (as prescribed), development of an individualized plan of care/functional maintenance program, and caregiver training for implementation – maximize an individual's skills to maintain the highest level of functional independence
* provide oral care before meals with a citric swab to increase salivation
* offer small frequent meals throughout the day
* offer high-calorie, high protein finger foods throughout the day to increase intake of calories
* offer water frequently throughout the day to increase hydration
* evaluate for appropriate positioning to expedite safe, effective swallow function & meal completion

(Curfman, 2005)

Encouraging Eating in the Early & Mid Stages of Dementia

In the early to mid stages of a person's dementia many things can develop which cause an eating problem for the individual. The sense of taste can change normally as an individual ages and is more pronounced in individuals with Alzheimer's disease and certain other dementias. Some forms of dementia can lead to an increased craving for sweets. Mealtimes can present many challenges. A person with dementia may have a poor appetite, loss of interest in food, may forget to eat or that they have already eaten. But on a more basic level, the individual may have differentiating between what is food and what isn't, as well as problems in knowing what to do with utensils and even what to do with the food. Here are some ways to assist the person to eat a nutritious meal:

1) Difficulty in Recognition: Mark plates and utensils so it is clear that they belong to the individual since some individuals affected by dementia have great difficulty in knowing which plate is theirs. Have the person sit in the same place for each meal so they can develop a sense of familiarity.

2) Locate a comfortable place to eat: Some individuals are not comfortable eating at a dining table – try to allow the person to eat where he/she is most comfortable with the plate and utensils at a good height for the person; have everything within reaching distance for the person; and attempt to have the person sitting upright in as close to the usual posture of sitting in a chair eating at a table.

3) Do not allow the person to eat alone: The person should not eat alone; some individuals forget to eat and need prompting (or reminders to eat); some individuals put food in their mouths and forget the food is there (a potential choking hazard); and some people do not realize the need to eat. Eating is a social activity in most areas of the country and eating with others helps a person with dementia stay connected with their community.

4) Distractions can hinder eating: Serve meals in a quiet place so that the person can focus on eating. Turn off the television, radio, or overhead paging system. If an individual is easily distracted, keep the table setting simple – remove flowers, centerpieces and condiments. Use only the utensils needed for the meal.

5) Encourage healthy snacking: Many elders with dementia develop an affinity for sweets. The taste buds change with aging but the ability to taste sweets is the last taste to be lost. Most caregivers will try to steer away from sweets because of concerns about proper nutrition but this can be used as an advantage: bake cookies with dried fruits and vegetables; oatmeal cookies have excellent fiber and oatmeal can be added to anything to aid in nutrition; pumpkin and squash can be used to make a bar cookie; and there are many high protein snacks that taste like sweets.

6) Make foods palatable: Monitor smells of foods to see if the person seems to get nauseated with certain odors. Check the food temperature because a person may eat better if the food is served at its appropriate temperature. Some individuals with dementia also have difficulty in telling if a food or beverage is too hot to eat or drink.

7) Overwhelmed by choices: For individuals who freeze when offered too many choices – serve only one or two foods at a time. For example, serve mashed potatoes followed by chicken tenders.

8) Enhance foods with spices: Due to the changes in an older person's taste buds, food preferences will change. The ability to taste salt usually is lost early and it may not be appropriate to add more salt to an older person's diet (adding salt may be contraindicated due to other disease processes) – so food may taste better when it is spiced up (which makes it more flavorful).

9) Control intake of snacks: Place snack foods and finger foods in one area of the kitchen, so that they are easy to find and make sure that available foods are nutritious. Apples, carrots, and celery sticks make excellent foods to leave out where individuals may help themselves to the nutritious snacks. Be cautious in the selection of the handy snack if a person does not chew thoroughly or easily chokes.

10) Helping differentiate between food and non-foods: Some people with dementia will find it difficult to tell what is edible and what isn't, which can result in eating napkins, artificial or plastic fruits, bar soap, cleaning supplies, or just about anything that can be placed in a person's mouth. This can potentially be very dangerous. Use the same cautions as you would with any dangerous material and consider child-locks on cabinets to prevent ingestion of hazardous materials.

11) Assist with handling of plates and utensils: As a person's dementia progresses, the individual may have difficulty in using knives, forks, spoons and cups – he/she may spill food, drop food or drinks, or have problems coordinating the use of utensils. As a person loses the ability to manipulate silverware, provide finger food as much as possible. Some foods, however, do not lend toward being eaten with fingers, so help by spooning it into a person's mouth may be needed. Put the person's hand on your hand with the spoon as you fed him/her. Cups can be a big problem – due to spills or because they may forget which end they are supposed to drink from – buy some kid cups with a heavy duty built-in straws or a sippy cup with large handles.

12) Dealing with hidden foods: Foods can sometimes disappear for an individual with dementia if the foods seem to run together – try using heavy plastic plates that have divided compartments and high sides or a lip on the edge so the food is visible and it is not accidentally shoved off the plate (and disappears for the person). Some individuals will also hide food with their personal effects. Leaving snacks out can become a problem, yet snack foods may still be in demand. But limiting the amount of snack foods left out is better. Observe where the person's favorite hiding spots are located and check them when food seems to disappear. Then it is simple to remove food and other inappropriate items the person may have hidden when the person is distracted.

13) Encourage adequate fluid intake: Don't overlook the importance of fluids. Water is essential to prevent dehydration and urinary tract infections. Adding liquid meal replacements and supplements such as Ensure or an instant breakfast to a person's meal is a wonderful way of adding calories as well as fluids, vitamins, and nutrients. (Water in tea or coffee is not a good substitute for plain water because these drinks have caffeine which can act as a diuretic and cause the person to urinate and worsen dehydration.) Have water available for the person to sip on and don't forget to encourage the person to drink plenty of water throughout the day.

14) Choking hazards: Avoid nuts, popcorn, hard candy, gum, and raw carrots for individuals who choke easily. These foods can get caught in the throat. Be alert for symptoms of choking and learn how to perform the Heimlich maneuver, just in case the person has problems.
(Alzheimer's Association, 2010; Knox, 2010)

Encourage Independence
(Do Not Encourage Dependence)

- **Make the most of the person's abilities.** Allow a person to eat from a bowl instead of a plate or use a plate with a lip around the edge, or allow a person to eat with a spoon instead of a fork – even with hands if it's easier.
- **Serve finger foods.** Chicken fingers, potato wedges, cheese cubes, cherry tomatoes, etc. are easier to pick up with hands and manipulate or eat on the go.
- **Demonstrate how to eat or use a "watch me" technique.** Offer a demonstration of how to eat: hold a spoon, and make the motion of eating or eat with the person and show the person how to eat by example.

- **Don't worry about neatness.** Let individuals feed themselves as much as possible. Consider getting plates with suction cups and no-spill glasses.

Many of the conditions causing a person's dementia can cause difficulty eating for individuals as their disease progresses. The following chart outlines some of the problems involved and why these problems occur.

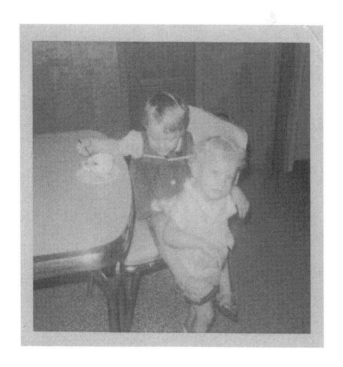

Eating Problems in the Different Dementias

Alzheimer's disease	Parkinson's disease	Frontotemporal dementia

■ Anosmia
  » diminished sense of smell
■ Ability to taste of food diminished
  » Prefers highly seasoned, spicy, & sweet foods because they are more satisfying
■ Food preferences change
■ Need to change consistency of food to enhance swallowing abilities
■ Easily distracted
  » May need prompting
	■ 50-63% of individuals with Parkinson's disease experience problems with eating at some point
	■ Oral
	  » Lingual tremor at rest
	  » Lingual tremor making the individual fatigued while eating as well as have problems swallowing
	  » Multiple lingual gestures during oral bolus manipulation & propulsion
	  » Need to change consistency of food to make easier to manage and swallow
	■ Pharyngeal
	  » Decreased laryngeal elevation
	  » Incomplete upper esophageal sphincter relaxation
	  » Pharyngeal residual after swallowing
	■ Esophageal
	  » Decreased muscle tone
		■ Increased appetite with increased sweet cravings
		■ Abnormal oral behaviors
		  » Atypical bite sizes
		  » Decreased chewing
		  » Eating non-edible things
		  » Involuntary bolus movement to the pharynx or into the unclosed airway before the elicitation of a swallow

Table Strategies for Managing Eating Problems
with Dementia and Dysphagia

FORGETFULNESS AND DISORIENTATION

UNABLE TO IDENTIFY THE SENSATION OF HUNGER AND THE NEED FOR FOOD

- Offer liquids and water consistently throughout the day – Dehydration may trigger increased combativeness and urinary tract infections, which can further the problems with eating
- Place beverage bars in places frequented by the person to encourage a person to drink more often

PLAYS WITH FOOD/FORGETS HOW TO EAT/DOES NOT RECOGNIZE FOOD – does not transition from the before-meal activity to the meal itself, thus continues to play with food because the person does not realize it is time to eat

- Offer environmental interventions to signal the change to eating, including altering the appearance of the table, such as using a tablecloth, flowers, baskets for napkins, and place mats

EATS WITH FINGERS INSTEAD OF UTENSILS

- Increase the number of finger foods being offered
- Serve hot cereal or soups in a mug, or cut fresh fruits and vegetables into bite-size pieces
- Offer portable items such as breakfast bars, finger gelatin, and 'edible containers' such as ice cream cones as options
- Continue to try to encourage eating with utensils if the individual's skill level can be advanced

DOES NOT USE UTENSILS CORRECTLY – Limit the number of utensils – Often individuals with dementia eat with a knife because it is picked up with the dominant hand to cut food [whether needed or not] and then the person forgets to put it down to select a fork or spoon

TOO MANY CHOICES – A person is unable to make choices if too much food or too many containers are present at one time
- Serve one course at a time so that the necessity of making choices is limited and there are fewer distractions
- When appropriate, allow menu selection and the choice between two or three main courses
- If dining at a restaurant, offer the menu and give the cueing needed to help with choices. For example, 'Would you prefer chicken or the meatloaf today?' If individuals cannot make choices at all and you know their food preferences, make suggestions, 'They have great chicken and dumplings here. Would you like to try the chicken and dumplings for lunch?'

OVERWHELMED BY TOO MUCH FOOD – If the person feels that there is too much food on their plate – use two plates, serving half a meal at a time

DEMONSTRATES AN INABILITY TO UNDERSTAND WHAT IS EXPECTED AT MEALTIME – Establish the same routine at each meal
- Reinforce with simple one-step directions using visual and gestural cueing
- Placement of the fork/spoon in the individual's preferred hand
- Hand-over-hand caregiver assistance may trigger the eating process

LIMITED ATTENTION SPAN – Has an inability to stay focused on the task of eating, limiting the meal from being consumed entirely
- Use simple concrete words
- Use touch and redirect the person to continue eating
- Offering five or six meals per day may be needed for individuals who are unable to eat much at any one time if they become agitated when caregivers attempt to refocus them

LEAVES THE TABLE DURING THE MEAL – The meal may be a combination of sitting and eating, followed by walking and eating finger foods from a bowl
- Make sandwiches with anything that will hold together
- Waist pouches may help someone who paces to keep their hands free so they can hold finger foods

JUDGMENT AND SAFETY

EATS FOOD PIECES THAT ARE TOO BIG TO SWALLOW SAFELY
- Assess food pieces for size, thickness, and consistency and make necessary adjustments
- Consider providing precut meats and other food items cut into bite-size pieces

EATS NONEDIBLES
- Avoid garnishes that are not easily chewed or eaten and those that are decorative in nature

POURS LIQUIDS ONTO FOODS
- Offer only food and when finished, offer water and fluids
- Place liquids in a container with a top and straw

TAKES ANOTHER PERSON'S FOOD
- Offer visual cueing for boundaries by using place mats to reduce interest in another's meal
- Square tables provide better definition of territory than round tables

Managing Perceptual Problems in Individuals with Dementia

VISION – Has difficulty discriminating boundaries between items
- Focus on color contrast in terms of the food to the plate or cup, and the contrast of the plate to the place mat (Supporting visual interpretation can reduce an individual's anxiety)
- Increase lighting in order to allow the person to see food better since older person's eyes need more lighting than a younger person's eyes

189

Managing Perceptual Problems in Individuals with Dementia
(continued)

- Monitor for glare – may need to use indirect light
- If a person has had a stroke or is visually impaired on one side – consider placing a person's plate more to the person's good side to so he/she may see the food better

COMMUNICATION – Understanding and being understood
- Develop a list of food preferences and dislikes
- Use sensory cueing with frequent gestures and pointing
- Remove a food or an item away from the table and then bring it back; or temporarily remove the food from the plate to regain attention
- Use verbal encouragement, such as, 'This really tastes good, would you please try it and tell me what you think?'
- When asking questions about food choices, use 'either/or' questions rather than 'yes/no' questions which could lead to no's and not eating

WEIGHT GAIN/LOSS
- Providing large meals or double servings at the meals the person eats the best such as breakfast may help to maintain weight
- Offer small frequent meals or snacks between meals and before bedtime
- Alternate hot and cold foods to help trigger swallowing
- Enhance food tastes – consider using honey and sugar to enhance the taste of foods, if medically appropriate – Sweet taste receptors remain intact through the end stage; therefore, residents with end-stage disease usually favor sweets and can be enticed to eat by adding sweet thickeners to foods
- Offer high-protein and high calorie foods

ANXIETY
- Sometimes individuals with dementia become obsessed about seating placement – may say someone is seated 'in my place' or

ANXIETY (continued)
  demand the same seat every time and will become aggressive if someone else sits 'in my seat' – Consider using name cards, or remove the resident's chair until just before the person arrives at the table
- Sits too close to others or someone he/she dislikes – Be aware of a person's preferred tablemates since an acceptable peer group is important to many individuals

CONCERNS AND PRIDE
- Delusions – Sometimes individuals with dementia have false beliefs: The person believes they have no money to pay for a meal: consider issuing meal tickets or 'credit cards'; have a bill filled out with a receipt that helps an individual with 'no money' to accept the meal and pay later
  » Offer colored play money for individuals to use, or tell them the meal is paid for by insurance
  » Inform them that the meal is part of the 'club' membership; therefore, it is required that the person eat dinner at the club

DINING AREA – environment & equipment
- Some individuals may behave disruptively because of room size and setup, type and size of tables, lighting, window glare, dishes, glassware, or utensils
  » Have a variety of tables available to meet specific, individualized needs
  » A table for one or two may be needed if an individual with dementia is experiencing hostility or paranoia
  » Square tables create a sense of 'my space'; round tables create the illusion of someone eating off another's plate
- Glare from windows or lights can create agitation; if feasible, encourage natural sunlight
- Provide cups and glassware that are easy to grasp
- Consider serving soups and hot cereals in a mug or soup bowl with handles

DINING AREA – environment & equipment (continued)
• Use special cups with large handles and built-in straws for individuals who spill a lot

(Alzheimer's Association, 2010)

Enteral Feeding and End-of-Life Decisions

As a person's dementia advances, nearly all of these individuals will decrease their intake of food and water. Use of feeding tubes in individuals with dementia is controversial and caregivers should be educated on the realistic expectations of the impact regarding the utilization of a feeding tube. Many people in the advanced stages of dementia have a feeding tube placed. A feeding tube is a tube inserted through the abdominal wall into the stomach known as a percutaneous gastrostomy tube or percutaneous endoscopic gastrostomy tube (PEG tube) or a tube inserted into the small intestine known as a jejunostomy tube (J tube). Fluids, liquid nutrition, and medications can be given to a person through these tubes.

Discussions surrounding feeding tubes being used to sustain life in the final stage of dementia should include the individual and family early in the person's disease, if possible, to determine what a person would wish be done when the illness advances to this stage. It is better to have the person's input while the person is able to state his/her own preference regarding feeding tube use after he/she has lost the ability to communicate. If the individual can no longer participate in the discussion, it is important to provide caregivers who are the decision makers for an individual with adequate information regarding available treatment options, what a feeding tube can and cannot do, and the consequences related to inserting a feeding tube or choosing not to place one as well as alternatives for nutritional intake (Curfman, 2005).

Insertion of a Feeding Tube

Feeding tubes are used on a long-term basis and are called percutaneous endoscopic gastrostomy tubes, or **PEG** tubes. Insertion of a PEG tube usually takes less than an hour and is done while the person is sedated. A small opening is made through the skin and the tube is inserted into the stomach. A PEG tube is inserted through this opening and secured in place.

Risks of the Procedure

Putting in a feeding tube is usually a simple procedure that does not cause serious or dangerous problems. There are several potential problems which could occur, including bleeding or perforation into the abdominal wall by the tube – this occurs in less than 10% of individuals. Issues which are common in use of a feeding tube for nutrition include infection at the site, leakage at the insertion site; nausea and vomiting which could lead to aspiration; and diarrhea from use of a liquid supplement. Long range problems include the tube becoming obstructed or being pulled out, or the tube becoming dislodged. Additional problems include infection at the site of tube insertion, as well as erosion into the intestinal wall (which would necessitate intervention).

What Can a Feeding Tube do?

It is important to define the overall goals of care and what a feeding tube can and cannot do. Some of the goals of using a feeding tube include improving a person's nutritional status, preventing aspiration, being able to give a person medications, and keeping the person comfortable. In individuals who have had a stroke and have a physiological dysphagia and in individuals with advanced Parkinson's disease who either fatigue easily or have issues with aspiration, feeding tubes can assist in hydration, nutrition, and lessening the occurence of aspiration. However, individuals with advanced dementia generally do not gain a significant amount of weight or have improved physical function when a feeding tube is placed. Feeding tubes also do not help wounds heal to a significant degree or prevent the occurrence of new pressure sores in individuals with advanced dementia (Ersek & Hanson, 2009).

Aspiration pneumonia is a common complication of a well-hydrated individual or in a person with a feeding tube who has excessive contents in their stomach and the person vomits or has some of the contents reflux up the esophagus and into the lungs. Aspiration can cause pneumonia and death in individuals with advanced dementia. And while prevention of aspiration is a goal of tube feeding, studies have shown that individuals with advanced dementia who have feeding tubes continue to aspirate at the same rate as before the tube was placed. Individuals who have a feeding tube placed are more likely to be hospitalized and have to go through painful procedures. Finally, people who have feeding tubes sometimes need their extremities forcefully restrained to keep the person from pulling out their feeding tube.

Will a Feeding Tube Prolong Life in Advanced Dementia?

The decision to use a feeding tube or not to use a feeding tube can be difficult. The answer to the question should be based on personal preference guided by available scientific evidence. Research indicates that there is no conclusive evidence on the benefits of feeding tubes in individuals with advanced dementia. Several studies have compared dementia patients with and without feeding tubes and most studies have found that a feeding tube does not prolong life for individuals with advanced dementia. Most individuals with feeding tubes do not survive very long; there are several studies which show that 20-30% of individuals who have feeding tubes die within a month after placement and 50-60% die within a year (Ersek & Hanson, 2009). Feedings tubes do extend life in individuals who have a mechanical problem with swallowing such as strokes, advanced Parkinson's disease, or neurodegenerative disorders who have severe muscle weakness affecting their swallowing.

Other Options for a Person with Dementia

If a person has decreased intake or has a decreased appetite caused by infection, constipation, or depression, then these conditions should be treated to see if the person's appetite improves. If a loss of appetite is caused by a side effect of a medication, then the medicine causing the problem may require a change if possible. If a person can still chew and swallow, caregivers may wish to continue to assist the person with eating and, if necessary, hand feed the person. Often, the diet is modified and a person is given foods that are easy to eat. One important benefit of hand feeding is that it is a time for caregivers and families to interact with a person with dementia. At this time, the person should be fed favorite foods so that eating is a pleasant experience for the person.

Even when people with late-stage dementia can no longer eat because of swallowing problems, the person may be able to take small tastes of their favorite foods and beverages. Excellent mouth care is important to maintain the person's oral hygiene and comfort. Other care includes treating pain and other symptoms, and providing emotional and spiritual support for the person and family. Many people with advanced dementia who cannot eat and drink qualify for hospice care, which can be provided in a home setting or a nursing home (Ersek & Hanson, 2009).

Chapter 7 References

Alzheimer's Association. (2010). Eating. Retrieved April 12, 2010 from http://www.alz.org/living_with_alzheimers_eating.asp

Bankhead, C. (2010). Old-Age vision problems linked to Dementia. MedPage Today. Retrieved April 17, 2010 from http://www.medpagetoday.com/Geriatrics/GeneralGeriatrics/18633

Curfman, S. (2005). Managing dysphagia in residents with dementia: skilled intervention for a common – and troubling – disorder. Nursing Homes. Retrieved 4-13-2010 from http://findarticles.com/p/articles/mi_m3830/is_8_54/ai_n15338409/

Curfman, S. (2010). Managing Dysphagia in Residents with Dementia: SKILLED INTERVENTION FOR A COMMON – AND TROUBLING – DISORDER. Nursing Homes/Long Term Care Management http://www.wrightstuff.biz/madyinrewide.html

Ersek, M., & Hanson, L. (2009). Tube Feeding Decisions for People with Advanced Dementia. AGS Foundation. Retrieved April 17, 2010 from http://www.healthinaging.org/public_education/pef/tube_feeding.php

How to Care. (2010). Eating and Nutrition. Retrieved April 18, 2010 from http://www.howtocare.com/diet2.htm

Knox, E. (2010). Tips on…Eating (Early and Middle Stages of Dementia). Retrieved April 12, 2010 from http://www.ec-online.net/knowledge/Articles/eatingtip1.html

MedLine Plus. (2010). Aging Changes to the Senses. Retrieved April 17, 2010 from http://www.nlm.nih.gov/medlineplus/ency/article/004013.htm

myDoc. (2010). Dementia and eating difficulties. Retrieved April 12, 2010 from http://www.mydr.com.au/seniors-health/dementia-and-eating-difficulties

SCIE. (2010) Eating well for people with dementia. Retrieved April 17, 2010 from http://www.scie.org.uk/publications/dementia/eating/environment.asp

Chapter 8

Sleepless Nights or UP ALL NIGHT AND ENERGY FROM NO-WHERE!

Individuals with dementia may experience a surge of energy in the night-time hours which can be problematic when these individuals are at great risk for falls and injury. There are many reasons why individuals suffering from dementia awaken through the night and there are many problems caused by a person not obtaining an appropriate amount of sleep. This chapter will discuss the biological processes occurring during sleep, the consequences of not getting an adequate amount of REM sleep, triggers which impair an older person's ability to sleep, and ways to increase length/ improve the quality of restful sleep in confused individuals. A brief discussion of Dream-Directed Behaviors will also be presented.

Introduction

Sleep disorders are a common problem for older adults in general and a significant source of concern for older individuals suffering from dementia. Sleep problems are often under-diagnosed and may result in problems affecting a person's overall health. Insomnia and other sleep problems are very bothersome in individuals suffering from dementia, who may be up all night long. Approximately 25% of adults with dementia experience sleep disturbances (Rose & Lorenz, 2010). The most common complaints are decreased night-time sleeping and increased daytime napping (Zec & Burkett, 2008). There are several diverse factors which may contribute to sleep disturbances in many older individuals related to changes associated with normal aging including lifestyle changes, retirement, health problems, death of relatives – spouse/family members, and changes in circadian rhythm. Changes in sleep patterns may be part of the normal aging process; however, many of these disturbances may be related to pathological processes that are not considered a normal part of aging including dementia (Brannon et al, 2009).

Insomnia affects a person's quality of life and can lead to excessive daytime sedation, fatigue, worsening of other chronic medical conditions, negative impacts on psychological status causing depression and/or anxiety, worsening of cognitive problems, and can worsen a person's overall health. Sleep disorders can even hasten a person's death. Treating sleep problems in individuals with dementia usually improves the overall health of the person, but care must be taken when using medications to affect sleep because they can cause problems in older individuals such as falls, orthostatic hypotension (fall in blood pressure when sitting upright abruptly or with standing), and worsening of confusion as well as other problems. Treatments for sleep disorders include behavioral modifications, relaxation techniques, sleep hygiene, sleep restriction, sleep deprivation for individuals who are napping during the daytime, light therapy, cognitive behavioral therapies, valerian, Tai Chi, yoga, meditation, acupuncture, acupressure, and possibly medications, both over-the-counter as well as prescription medications (Brannon et al, 2009). To better understand how sleep affects health, the following discussion provides a brief review of the stages of sleep and how lack of sleep affects the chemical balance within a person's body.

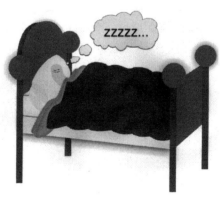

Sleep Patterns

Normal sleep is organized into four different stages that cycle throughout the night.

- Non-Rapid Eye Movement (Non-REM) sleep
  - Non-REM sleep is subdivided into 4 stages:
    - » Stages 1 and 2 – light sleep
    - » Stages 3 and 4 – deep sleep or slow-wave sleep (SWS)
  - With aging, an increase in the duration of stage 1 sleep and an increase in the number of shifts into stage 1 sleep occurs
  - Stages 3 and 4 decrease markedly with age, and, after 90 years – stages 3 and 4 may disappear completely
- Rapid Eye Movement (REM) sleep
  - Rapid eye movement (REM) sleep is the stage of sleep during which muscle tone decreases markedly; this stage is associated with bursts of dreaming
    - » Relative amounts of REM sleep are maintained until extreme old age, when most older adults show some decline in obtaining REM sleep

Need for Sleep as an Individual Ages

- Time in bed: increased time to go to sleep – older individuals spend more time lying in bed at night without attempting to sleep (reading, watching television, or eating in bed) or unsuccessfully trying to sleep
- Total sleep period: The time from sleep onset to the final awakening from the main sleep period of the day – total sleep period increases with age because of the increase in the number of night-time awakenings
- Total sleep time: The total sleep period minus the time spent awake during the sleep period is either reduced or unchanged in the older population compared with a younger age groups

- Sleep latency: The time from the decision to sleep to the onset of sleep. In women, sleep latency has been related to age increase in adults and hypnotic drug use, which decreases sleep latency
- Wake after sleep onset: The time spent awake from sleep onset to final awakening. An increase occurs in the time spent awake after sleep onset in older individuals. There are a number of reasons older individuals awaken through the night – need to void (bladder distention, urinary urgency), pain caused by arthritis, restless leg syndrome, and sleep apnea or dyspnea
- Sleep efficiency: is decreased due to nocturnal awakenings

(Brannon et al, 2009)

Older individuals spend more time in bed to get the same amount of sleep they obtained when they were younger; however, the total sleep time is slightly decreased with an increase in nocturnal awakenings and daytime napping. Older people have been observed to be more easily aroused from sleep by auditory stimuli (sounds), suggesting increased senstivity to environmental stimulation (Brannon, 2009). Often, older individuals tend to have earlier daytime somnelence and fatigue, which are not part of normal aging.

How the Effects of Aging Affect Sleep

- ➢ More alert in early morning
- ➢ Drowsier in early evening
- ➢ Less REM sleep
- ➢ Less eye movement density while asleep
- ➢ The cumulative effect of sleep deprivation leads to higher evening cortisol levels resulting in:
  - ○ Increased sleep fragmentation
  - ○ Increased Insulin resistance
  - ○ Encourages/hastens hippocampal atrophy
  - ○ Encourages deficits in hippocampus – which impairs learning & memory

---

Cortisol & Insomnia

Sleep is the time when a person's body renews and rejuvenates itself. It is a time of rebalancing, detoxification, and the re-booting of an individual's immune system. There are potentially serious long-term effects of sleep deprivation or insomnia including worsening of diabetes, heart disease, and cancers. Cortisol is a natural hormone which can be affected by sleep (or lack of sleep) and has anti-inflammatory properties; it is produced during the day and prevents natural cell repair from occurring; it is a steroid that is vital in the 'fight or flight' response to stress; and it is necessary, even for normal daily living. Without cortisol a person would not have the energy even to function but if cortisol levels are too high, it can result in health issues or even insomnia – becoming a problem which feeds upon itself i.e., insomnia causes higher cortisol levels and higher cortisol levels can lead to insomnia. When a person sleeps, cortisol levels are lowered and melatonin levels increase, allowing normal growth and repair of cells to occur. Without lowering cortisol levels, a person has more health problems, more weight gain, slower wound healing, more fatigue, and problems with learning and memory (Health Guide, 2010).

Other Health Problems & Insomnia

Individuals who sleep fewer than five hours a night are five times more likely to suffer hypertension than people who sleep well, according to a major study that highlights the concerns over links between sleep problems and serious illness (Medical News Today, 2008)

Diabetics are more likely to have poorly controlled glucose levels when they obtain less than five hours of uninterrupted sleep (Black, 2010)

Even though physically equal in fitness, obtaining less than 5 hours of sleep on a chronic basis made individuals physically weaker, have a significantly reduced exercise capacity, and a perceived greater effort during exercise (Fulcher & White, 2000)

Factors Affecting Sleep

- Chronic condition (% of population with this problem)
    - Hypertension (47%)
    - Arthritis (46%)
    - Enlarged prostate (22% of men)
    - Heart disease (18%)
    - Depression (16%)
    - Diabetes Mellitus (15%)
- Sleep Disordered Breathing
    - Snoring
    - Apnea
- Menopausal Women (causing a decline in endocrine physiology and greater reduction in slow-wave activity in non REM sleep)
- Restless Leg Syndrome (often the individual has a family member with this problem, can be secondary to iron deficiency or uremia, and can be exacerbated by antidepressants, caffeine, nicotine, alcohol, & inactivity)
- Medication use
- Nocturia: 65% of older adults experience needing to void during night-time sleep
- Neuropsychological impairment

Sundowning

Sundowning involves the occurrence or increase in occurrence of one or more abnormal behaviors in the late afternoon and evening hours which may continue into the night. A person who is experiencing sundowning may exhibit increased confusion, delusions, paranoia, hallucinations, and mood swings. They may become abnormally demanding, suspicious, and become upset or more disoriented. Sundowning is estimated to occur in 45% of persons diagnosed with Alzheimer's disease (Wikipedia, 2010). Wandering often occurs in individuals who are sundowning and is the second most common type of disruptive behavior in institutionalized persons with dementia. The danger involved in night-time wandering is a person becoming lost, often referred to as elopement. The cause of sundowning is unknown, but may be related to disturbed circadian rhythm. Another suspected cause is an adrenalin surge most individuals experience in the afternoon and evening hours throughout their adult lives, when this burst of energy is necessary to complete the day's tasks at the end of the day (getting off work, preparing dinner, bathing children, and getting ready for the next day). A person's body became accustomed to this adrenalin surge but, as an individual becomes older, and no longer has tasks to perform, the body does not recognize this fact and continues to produce an adrenalin surge. Confused individuals now have excessive energy and feel a need to do 'something' and thus wander or exhibit restless behaviors.

When the Sun Goes Down, the Night can be Terrifying

Individuals suffering from dementia may do well in the daytime but have problems in the afternoon and night-time hours. The dark can be a terrifying for individuals who are sent into a state of confusion when they are tired and less able to compensate. Some individuals are terrified by the shadows that occur in the dark, some may not know where they are or who they are with, and others may have visual as well as auditory hallucinations. A person may wonder who might know they are alone and if someone will break into their house and rob them – or worse. Whether the causes of night-time fears are physical, psychological or related to a disease such as Alzheimer's disease or another dementia, caregivers have found that night-time can be very frightening for a large number of these individuals – especially those who live alone (Senior Care, 2010). Many problems that occur at night with seniors are rooted in physical changes that result from normal aging changes to sensory input caused by decreased vision and hearing, as well as mobility changes due to arthritis or other medical conditions. Some night-time fears are connected to sleep disorders.

Companionship is one of the most important ways to manage night-time fears and the problems which accompany them – having someone stay with the person suffering from dementia can assist in promoting safety as well as help ensure the person's well-being. And this creates a caregiver, whether the caregiver is a family member or friend who comes to live with the person, the ill person comes to live with the caregiver, or the ill person moves to a facility which provides care for the person.

Dream Directed Behaviors

Another problem which can affect a person's ability to sleep is Dream Directed Behaviors. Normally when a person is sleeping and dreaming, the muscles are essentially paralyzed, preventing a person from acting out their dreams. But in this disorder, there is an abnormality occurring in the phase of REM sleep leading to movement during dreams, which is referred to as Dream Directed Behavior (DDB). A person is able to carry out the activities in their dreams and can become violent and/or potentially cause injury to themselves or others. The behaviors are not directed at anyone or anything in particular though it may be that the person is enacting movements such as punching and kicking as well as leaps and even jumps in their bed during sleep (Sleep Disorders, 2010). It occurs after the 6th decade and occurs more commonly in men than women.

Some of the things that can protect a person who suffers from DDB disorder from harm include removing dangerous objects from their bedrooms, clearing furniture and other objects that can cause harm and making sure the person cannot wander away. Consider having the person sleep on the mattress on the floor or with cushions around their beds. For individuals who have frequent problems falling out of bed, a rail (such as a side-rail on a hospital bed or a toddler rail on the side of the bed) to prevent the person from jumping out of bed may prevent injury. Loose rugs should have double-sided tape to prevent a person from slipping and falling and one should ensure that a person has grippers on the bottoms of the socks if they wear them to bed.

Sometimes, DDB disorder requires medications but caution should be used because medications for insomnia can worsen this problem and cause falls in older individuals. Clonazepam has been found to be very effective in treating these disorders and in fact, success rates have been reported as being extremely high (Sleep Disorders, 2010).

Enhancing Sleep

Improving sleep habits must include establishing a bedtime routine, enhancing the sleep environment, and, if necessary, reducing daytime napping. Medications may be necessary but other facotrs must always be considered. To create an inviting sleeping environment and promote rest for a person with dementia:

- Maintain a regular routine including times for meals and for going to bed as well as getting up
- Sunlight exposure
- Encourage regular exercise, but not within three hours before bedtime
- Avoid alcohol, caffeine and nicotine
- Treat pain
- If a person is taking a cholinesterase inhibitor (tacrine, donepezil, rivastigmine or galantamine), monitor if the medication seems to make the person sleepy – then give at bedtime; or if the medication stimulates the person the person – then give the medication in the morning
- Make sure the bedroom temperature is comfortable i.e., if the room is too warm, it can make it difficult to sleep
- Provide nightlights and keep the room free of clutter to prevent injury [if the person gets out of bed at night]
- If the person awakens, discourage staying in bed while awake i.e., use the bed only for sleep – do not eat in bed, watch television in bed, or read in bed

Enhancing Sleep in Individuals with Dementia

- Arrange a medical check-up to identify and treat physical symptoms
- Treat pain with an analgesic at bedtime
- Screen for depression – treatment may be necessary
- Consider the possible side effects of medications that may cause sleep problems
- Consider environmental factors

Environmental Causes of Sleep Problems in Individuals with Dementia

Sleeping problems may be caused by environmental causes including:

- The room being too hot or too cold – a cooler room is more conducive to sleep
- Poor lighting may cause disorientation or hallucinations (which are caused by shadows)
- The person may need to urinate and may not be able to find the bathroom
- Changes in the environment can cause disorientation and confusion
- Changes in routine can cause problems sleeping

Things to Try

- Keep the environment as consistent as possible – consistent bedtimes and bedtime rituals
- Check whether the person is too hot or too cold since dementia can affect a person's internal thermostat
- Shadows, glare or poor lighting may contribute to agitation and hallucinations, so provide nightlights to diminish shadows
- Nightlights may help cut down on confusion at night and may assist the person to find the bathroom
- Make sure the bed and bedroom are comfortable and familiar (familiar objects may help to orient a confused person)

208

- Avoid having daytime clothing in view at night, as this may cause confusion and make the person think it is time to get up
- Make sure that the person is getting adequate exercise (try taking walks each day to burn up pent up energy)

Other Causes of Insomnia

- Going to bed too early
- Daytime napping
- Overtiredness, causing tenseness and inability to fall asleep
- Too much energy – insufficient exercise so that the person does not feel tired
- Too much caffeine or alcohol
- Feeling hungry
- Agitation following an upsetting situation
- Disturbing dreams

Food and Drink

- Cut down on or eliminate use of caffeine (coffee, cola, tea, chocolate) during the day and cut out altogether after 3pm
- Cut down on or eliminate use of alcohol and/or tobacco
- If the person may be hungry at night, try a light snack just before bed or when they wake up, but encourage the person to stay sitting upright for at least 30 minutes after eating
- Herbal teas and warm milk may be helpful

Daily Routines

- Avoid any activities that may be upsetting to the person in the late afternoon
- If the person refuses to go to bed, try offering alternatives such as sleeping on the sofa or in a recliner
- If the person wanders at night, consider allowing this but make sure the environment is safe
- Try a back rub before bed or during wakeful period

- Try playing soft music beside the bed or use background noise devices
- Gently remind the person that it is night-time and time for sleep

Other Considerations

Problems with sleeping or late evening agitation are often a stage in dementia that is bothersome, difficult to manage, and potentially dangerous if the person falls or wanders outside at night. Many individuals with dementia sleep more during the advanced stages of their illness. Sleep problems are among the most difficult symptoms of dementia for caregivers, who must be able to get adequate sleep themselves. (Better Health Channel, 2010)

Medications for Sleep Changes

In some cases, when non-drug approaches fail to work or the sleep changes are accompanied by disruptive night-time behaviors, medications may be necessary. Experts recommend that medication treatment follow geriatric prescribing guidelines: 'begin low and go slow' i.e., use the smallest effective dose possible, give the medication an adequate amount of time to work, increase a medication only when necessary and only increase in small increments, and only use the medication when necessary – weaning and removing it when possible. There are risks associated with the use of medications for sleep problems in older individuals who are cognitively impaired including worsening confusion and agitation, increased risk for falls and fractures, and a decline in the ability to perform the activities of daily living. If sleep medications are used, it is discouraged to use them on a long-term basis and an attempt should be made to discontinue them after a regular sleep pattern has been established (Alzheimer's Association-Treatment for Sleep, 2010). The type of medication prescribed is often influenced by behaviors that may accompany the sleep changes.

Types of Medications Used to Treat Sleep Problems

Alzheimer's medications are not indicated for insomnia but individuals taking these agents have been shown to sleep better:

- N-Methyl D – Aspartate Receptor Antagonist (NMDA)
  - ○ Approved to treat moderate to severe AD
  - ○ Blocks NMDA receptors which help regulate glutamate; assists in calming sundowning and night-time behaviors
    - » Memantine HCL (Namenda): 5mg daily at bedtime for 1 week, then 5mg twice a day for 1 week, then 5mg in the morning & 10 mg at bedtime for 1 week, then 10 mg twice a day

- Cholinesterase inhibitors
  - ○ Donazepril HCl (Aricept): 5 mg once a day for 1 month then 10 mg once a day
  - ○ Ravistigmine (Exelon): begin at 1.5mg twice a day, increase every 2 weeks until the optimal dose is reached – usually 6 mg twice a day (maximum dose is 12 mg a day); Also available in a patch used once a day (dose-4.6mg/24 hours & 9.5 mg/24 hours) – excellent for individuals who are unable to take medications by mouth or who refuse to take medications
  - ○ Galantamine (Galantamin): 4mg twice a day; increase every 4 weeks until optimal dose is reached (maximum dose is 12 mg twice a day)

Sleeping Medications

Nonbenzodiazepines – some are indicated for sleep and some are indicated for anxiety management – all have a side effect of somnelence

- Alprazolam (Xanax) 0.5 to 1 mg only as needed
- Clonazepam (Klonipin) 0.5 to 1 mg only as needed
- Eszopiclone (Lunesta): 1, 2, or 3 mg at bedtime only as needed
- Lorazepam (Ativan) 0.5 to 1 mg only as needed
- Zaleplon (Sonata): 5, 10, or 20 mg at bedtime only as needed
- Zolpidem (Ambien): 5 to10 mg at bedtime only as needed

Benzodiazepines (can be hazardous in elders due to potential for falls, worsening of confusion, delusions, and hallucinations as well as potentially increasing agitation)

- Temazepam (Restoril): 7.5 to 15mg at bedtime only as needed
- Triazolam (Halcion): 0.125mg to 0.25mg at bedtime only as needed

Melatonin receptor agonists

- Ramelteon (Rozerem): 8 mg at bedtime only as needed

Sedating **Antidepressants** are not indicated to treat insomnia but have assisted in enhancing sleep in individuals with dementia

- Citalopram (Celexa): 10-40 mg once a day
- Duloxetine (Cymbalta): 20-60 mg once a day
- Escitalopram (Lexapro): 5-20 mg once a day
- Paroxetine (Paxil): 10-40 mg once a day
- Paroxetine CR (Paxil CR): 12.5-37.5 mg once a day
- Sertraline (Zoloft): 25-50 mg once a day

Antihistamines are commonly found in over-the-counter sleeping medications. They are dangerous in older individuals with or without dementia because they can cause worsening of confusion, delusions and hallucinations, and increase the incidence of falls – use cautiously

- Diphenhydramine (Benadryl): 12.5 to 25 mg at bedtime only as needed

Antihistamines (continued)
- Hydroxizine (Atarax): 12.5 to 25 mg at bedtime only as needed
- Meclizine (Antivert): 12.5 to 25 mg at bedtime only as needed

Antiseizure agents are not indicated for treating insomnia in individuals with dementia but have been used to manage behavioral problems and have a side effect of causing sleepiness – if a person is taking this medication, dose at bedtime
- Divalproic Acid (Depakote): 125-500 mg once a day at bedtime or twice a day

Antipsychotic medications are not indicated to treat behavioral problems in individuals with dementia nor for treating insomnia but they are sometimes used when night-time behaviors are potentially dangerous for the person or others (use with caution and wean off the medication when able if possible – see section on potential side effects and how to monitor the safety of the person taking an antipsychotic medication)
- Aripiprazole (Abilify): 2-30 mg once a day or twice a day
- Olanzapine (Zyprexa): 1.25-10 mg at bedtime or twice a day
- Quetiapine (Seroquel): 12.5-200 mg at bedtime or twice a day
- Risperidone (Risperdal): 0.25 to 3 mg at bedtime or twice a day
- Ziprasidone (Geodon): 20-80 mg once a day or twice a day

Anxiolytic agents are not indicated for sleep in individuals with dementia but have been used when a person is agitated and will not calm down to go to sleep
- Alprazolam (Xanax): 0.25-0.5 mg only as needed
- Clonazepam (Klonipin): 0.125-2 mg only as needed
- Clorazepapte (Tranxene): 3.75-15 mg only as needed
- Lorazepam (Ativan): 0.5 to 2mg only as needed

(Fragoso & Gill, 2007; Beers list, 2006; Mayhew, 2001; Monthly Prescribing Reference (MPR), 2010; Sleepdex, 2010)

Chapter 8 References

Alzheimer's Association. (2010). Treatment for Sleep. Retrieved March 25 from http://www.alz.org/alzheimers_disease_10429.asp

Better Health Channel. (2010). Dementia and sleeping problems. Retrieved April 17, 2010 from http://www.betterhealth.vic.gov.au/bhcv2/bhcarticles.nsf/pages/Dementia_and_sleeping_problems

Black, E. (2010). Diabetes and Insomnia. Quality Health. Retrieved April 18, 2010 from http://www.qualityhealth.com/diabetes-articles/diabetes-insomnia

Brannon, G., Vij, S., & Gentili, A. (2009). Sleep Disorder, Geriatric. eMedicine from WebMD. Retrieved April 17, 2010 from http://emedicine.medscape.com/article/292498-overview

Fragoso, C., & Gill, T. (2007). Sleep Complaints in Community-Living Older Persons: A Multifactorial Geriatric Syndrome. *Journal of the American Geriatric Society.* 55(11); 1853-1866.

Fulcher, K., & White, P. (2000). Strength and physiological response to exercise in patients with chronic fatigue syndrome. *Journal of Neurology, Neurosurgery & Psychiatry* 2000; 69:302-307.

Health Guide. (2010). Effects Of Insomnia The Health Problems A Lack Of Sleep Can Cause. Retrieved April 18, 2010 from http://www.fqwz.com/2010/03/health-guide-effects-of-insomnia-the-health-problems-a-lack-of-sleep-can-cause

Kalapatapu, R. & Schimming, C. (2009). Update on neuropsychiatric symptoms of dementia: Antipsychotic use. *Geriatrics.* 64 (5). 10-18.

Mayhew, M. (2001). How should I manage insomnia in the Elderly? Medscape for Nurses. Retrieved April 18, 2010 from http://www.medscape.com/viewarticle/413367

Medical News Today. (2008). Insomnia linked to Hypertension. Retrieved April 18, 2010 from http://www. medicalnewstoday.com/articles/112213.php

Monthly Prescribing Reference (MPR). (2010). Haymarket Media: New York, NY.

Rose, K. & Lorenz, R. (2010). Sleep disturbances in dementia. *Journal of Gerontological Nursing.* 36(5). 9-14.

Senior Journal. (2006) Beers Criteria for mediations to avoid in the elderly. Retrieved October 14, 2006 from http:// seniorjournal.com/NEWS/Eldercare/3-12-08Beers.htm

Sleepdex. (2010). Sleep aides for seniors. Retrieved April 18, 2010 from http://www.sleepdex.org/senior-meds.htm

Sleep Disorders (2010). What Causes REM Sleep Behavior Disorder? Retrieved April 18, 2010 from http:// apneasleepdisorders.com/what-causes-rem-sleep-behavior-disorder

Zec, & Burkett. (2008). Non-pharmacological and pharmacological treatment of the cognitive and behavioral symptoms of Alzheimer's disease. *Journal of NeuroRehabilitation.* (23). 425-438.

Chapter 9

Family Issues

Family members experience many different reactions to a loved one's diagnosis of dementia. Emotions, family dynamics, and family members' levels of understanding affect acceptance of the disease and impact family reactions. Difficult decisions will be made. Family conflict can occur. Feelings of anxiety, frustration, depression, and loss of control are normal and can create problems for caregivers. This chapter will discuss the emotional issues occurring when a family member receives a diagnosis of dementia, role changes which occur, family conflict, and strategies to manage family issues.

Introduction

The daughter arrives home after a trip to the grocery store and she is unable to locate her Dad. She searches his usual spots including his room, the bathroom, the backyard, and the kitchen – yet she cannot locate him. She begins to worry and asks neighbors if anyone has seen him – No Luck: No one has seen Dad. She calls her sister who has not spoken with Dad today.

She gets in her car and drives around the neighborhood. She drives around for 2 hours without locating Dad. She goes back home to call the police who tell her he must be missing for 48 hours before he is officially a missing person.

This not an uncommon problem when a confused individual wanders off.

The problem of dementia affects every family member but most impacts the immediate caregiver who must contend daily with difficult issues including wandering, aggressive behaviors, and a variety of other problems. This is in addition to managing the activities of daily living such as eating, grooming, administering medications, and daily life.

Every individual suffering from dementia is a member of a family and every member of that family unit is affected by the illness in some manner. When a loved one is diagnosed with any type of dementia, including Alzheimer's disease, the effects on the family can be overwhelming. The reality that someone you love has a devastating illness that will progress to the point where the individual is no longer the person you once knew – this can trigger a range of emotions including fear, sadness, confusion and anger. Conflicts are common as family members struggle to deal with the situation.

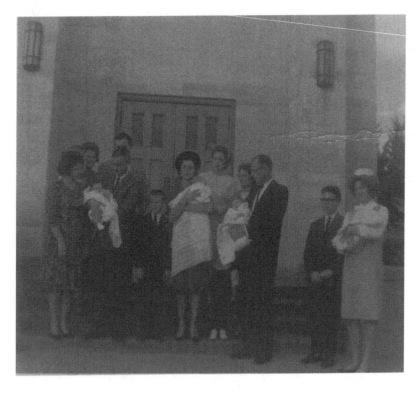

Issues Caregivers May Face in Caring for an Individual with a Diagnosis of Dementia

---

Wants all the caregiver's time and attention

Makes constant unreasonable demands

Is inflexible, critical, or negative

Unable to manage bills and finances but refuses to allow anyone to assist

Refuses to take medications

Complains about real or imagined physical symptoms

Acts normal and charming in front of others but inappropriate at home

Exhibits bizarre or inappropriate behaviors

Has become suspicious or paranoid

Experiences increasing memory loss

Exaggerates or 'cries wolf'

Prefers to stay in bed and 'wait to die'

Refuses to allow others to assist with care

Becomes furious when something does not go as the person wishes

Gets mad when told 'No'

Wants to eat constantly, not eat at all, or wants to eat only one thing

Refuses to take showers or change soiled clothing

Many family members report experiencing frustration, resentment, grief and loss of intimacy while at the same time increasing protectiveness and tenderness towards the person for whom they are caring. Spouses may begin to mourn the loss of their partner, including loss of intimacy with their partners, as roles shift from marital to caregiving (Health Central, 2010).

219

Family Issues

Many families are reluctant to seek help until a crisis arises, which may then force the family to seek outside sources. Research has shown that it can take some families up to two years before asking for that outside help (HealthCentral.com, 2010). Initially, there seems to be a strong desire to go on as if everything is the same, to stick with familiar routines as much as possible, and to deny that there is an issue.

The role change for caregivers begins when at least one daily task needs to be done for the person with a diagnosis of dementia – a reminder to take a shower or to change one's clothes. Many family members may begin to take on more responsibilities – many of which they had not done before, such as wife balancing the checkbook, a duty that once was the husband's responsibility, and a husband taking on housekeeping tasks such as doing laundry and cooking. The early stage of caregiving is marked by many struggles with identifying the problems, altering day-to-day life to accommodate a person's declining abilities, and negotiating decision-making – which may not be a smooth process.

Family Issues

- A wife who refuses to share information on her husband's physical health and mental abilities
- The family who refuses to accept the diagnosis of a dementing illness
- The sister who arrives from out-of-town who wishes to dictate the way care is directed
- The son who visits once every 3 years and accuses the nursing home staff of neglect and mistreatment
- The relatives who argue during a time of crisis

Family members experience many different reactions as they interact with caregivers and other family members. Emotions and intelligence are factors which affect how individuals deal with a diagnosis of dementia for a loved one. Difficult decisions are made that will profoundly affect the person with dementia and the family. In the face of these stressful situations, caregivers may become aware of strong feelings or may notice changes in their own behavior and activities. Or they may not be aware and react strongly. Feelings of anxiety, frustration, depression, and loss of control are normal and natural responses to these types of difficult situations.

Depression & Anxiety

Depression is common for families caring for a person with a diagnosis of dementia. Sometimes caregivers feel sorry for themselves, while at other moments their sadness is for the person with the disease. Caregivers may experience a lack of energy which is needed to socialize or pursue activities that were once meaningful. In response to the new emotional and physical demands, caregivers may have changes in appetite or sleep habits as well as worry about what the future holds.

Anger

Anger can periodically emerge. Family members may wonder how they can feel angry with someone they love who is sick. Frustration and anger in this kind of situation are common and normal. Sometimes families blame the person with dementia for acting inappropriately – not realizing the behaviors are a result of a physical disease affecting the brain, not realizing the person's abilities are declining, and not realizing the person cannot remember. The individual with dementia may seem 'normal' at times and at other times, there may be a lack of control of impulses and families may be unable to rationalize or reason with the person. A person with a diagnosis of dementia may exhibit irritating behavior, seem ungrateful for the care that is provided, or be difficult to manage. Family members, particularly spouses, may feel deserted at a time in life when companionship seems very important.

Guilt

Guilt may be in response to these conflicting feelings and previous beliefs, values, and experiences. Family members may wonder if they are doing enough, have done everything possible for the person, or are making the right decisions in care. Guilt may arise over misunderstandings that one family member had with the person in the past or with other family members.

Uncertainty

Families must recognize that any close relationship that endures over time will have many aspects. An illness can create stress which touches every member of the family but will affect each family member differently. Only one thing is certain – new emotions usually occur and these changes are normal. Reaching out for help will assist families to cope and remain intact.

Role Changes
Adjusting to new roles

Every person plays a role in families, communities, and societies. The role of an individual is the basis for all human relationships and interactions. Many grow comfortable in their roles and come to depend on others for fulfilling the roles that they play. In a family, people learn to rely on each other for certain things: a family may look to grandma to organize and make preparations for the large holiday gatherings; a wife may count on her husband to manage finances and pay bills; or a grown son still turns to his aging parents for advice and emotional support. Intellectual, behavioral, or emotional changes that accompany a diagnosis of dementia can alter individuals' abilities to function in their accustomed roles. Families must be cognizant that these changes occur and make adjustments accordingly.

Feelings of loss

Feelings of loss commonly occur for a person with a diagnosis of dementia and family members who are experiencing role changes. For individuals who have been accustomed to making decisions and managing personal and financial affairs, the realization that someone else is making decisions and that others are now called upon to perform certain tasks may be upsetting. Family members and caregivers who must learn to assume different responsibilities, they may be anxious, angry, or sad about the situation. Sometimes cognitive impairment caused by a dementia makes it impractical for a person to continue working, resulting in an unplanned and early retirement as well as financial strain. A person with a diagnosis of dementia and his/her family experience many adjustments and changes as well as a mixture of emotions including sadness, anger, and anxiety. Families must cope with many losses and should work to create effective strategies that compensate for these losses of abilities, independence, function, and thinking as well as the eventual loss of the ill person.

Intimacy: Sexual functioning

Sexual relationships also change. The person with a diagnosis of dementia may no longer desire sexual contact while a healthy spouse must struggle with feelings of rejection, anger and frustration. Some may experience an increased sexual desire and make excessive demands for frequent sexual encounters. On the other hand, the healthy spouse may no longer feel sexually attracted to the person suffering from dementia and may experience feelings of guilt. The caregiving role becomes more one of a parent than a partner and can result in a change in the nature of intimacy. Emotional bonding and friendship may undergo changes as the person's behavior changes. Caregivers may also feel that the person with a diagnosis of dementia is selfish and unappreciative, which can cause further emotional issues.

Difficulties in Social Situations

Embarrassment

Families may attempt to protect the person with a diagnosis of dementia in social situations. Families may try to compensate or 'cover up' for the person's forgetfulness, changing behaviors, or diminished social skills. Filling in missing words for the person or diverting the focus of attention away are common maneuvers of caregivers. Experiencing a sense of discomfort or embarrassment is normal and deciding what to tell friends and acquaintances can become difficult.

Isolation

Is it best to isolate a person so a difficult situation is avoided? Should the person with a diagnosis of dementia and his/her family continue with their social lives as if nothing had changed? There are no easy answers. Some situations may now be more stressful than others. The goal is to keep the person as socially active as possible – being attentive to physical safety and psychological safety of others, including children within the family. Social isolation of a person with dementia may lead to a lower level of functioning and/or increased confusion.

Effects on the Healthy Spouse

Spouses of individuals with a diagnosis of dementia must face some alterations in their social worlds. Healthy spouses may realize that some acquaintances visit less frequently, they may no longer enjoy going out on weekends to a play or movie, or the spouse may be less affectionate. Disrupting the person's routine or frequent travel to new places can be upsetting and is often discouraged. Each spouse must develop a comfortable strategy suitable for their particular circumstance in order to meet the continuing needs of the healthy spouse for social involvement, which is also important. If it is not appropriate for the person with dementia to continue certain activities, the spouse does not have to sacrifice totally – changes can be made to meet the emotional and social needs of the spouse or caregiver. Friends or family members can join the caregiver for an occasional outing. Arrangements may be made to have someone stay with the person with dementia to allow caregivers time away to meet their own needs. Every person requires time for work and time for leisure, particularly the caregiver of the person with a diagnosis of dementia. 'Breaks' or periods of time away from the person with dementia can re-energize caregivers, allowing them to continue caring for the ill person.

Sharing the burden

Altering social life can be one of the most difficult issues for family members to manage after a diagnosis of dementia. Lost social abilities may make those who love the ill person feel the saddest. This is understandable since the way people grow to love one another is largely based on the person's social traits – sense of humor, kindness, and special interests. Those who are closest may experience a strong mixture of feelings as changes occur in these areas. Talking with family or friends, support groups, and professionals about the impact of these alterations may help. Families and friends may draw together to provide mutual support or may become divided, depending on each individual's stage of understanding and acceptance. Many experience a grieving process over the loss of the person they once knew even before the physical death occurs. Support and being able to vent frustration as well as sadness can ease the burden. And when the responsibility of care is shared, tasks may be much more bearable.

To Tell or Not to Tell

The Dilemma: Telling others

Sometimes people choose not to tell others because they are embarrassed by the disease or by their symptoms. They hide problems in memory and other areas by avoiding social engagements. Another issue is the belief that friends and family would label them or treat them as 'less than' equal or the belief that friends and family would 'fall apart' if they knew. So they keep the disease a secret to spare others the burden of knowing.

Deciding not to tell

Trying to keep the disease a secret requires a great deal of effort and may result in stress to the person or the caregiver. Others who interact with the person are aware of problems, but are unsure of how to respond. Discussing the situation openly reduces stress and anxiety for all involved – the person with a diagnosis of dementia, family, and friends.

Children

Young children may need to know that a person's behavior is not a reflection of anything they have done. If children understand that a grandparent is sick, they are less likely to believe that the grandparent does not remember their names because he does not love them. If a caregiver wishes to enlist the aid of friends and neighbors, they can be more helpful once they have a clear understanding of the problem. In new social situations, everyone may feel more relaxed if they understand ahead of time about the person's difficulties and how they can make the situation most comfortable.

How to tell

Another issue that confronts families is how to explain the person's illness to others. A young child may not understand why his grandparent does not recognize him. Friends may be confused about why the person and his wife no longer go to social gatherings. Some friends and family members have trouble viewing the person as sick since they often appear physically healthy. The explanation of the illness that one gives will vary; there are no 'right' or 'wrong' answers – the best answer will vary from one situation to the next and may vary from one family to the next. Some families feel it is important to emphasize that the person has a neurological illness and not a mental or emotional disorder. In general, the best method is to be truthful and give a simple explanation. (NW, 2010)

Thinking About the Future

As the person with a diagnosis of dementia becomes more disabled, independent living, even with a caregiver, may become more difficult. Making the decision to move to a different setting such as a nursing home requires time and considerable planning. But this may ultimately be a reasonable solution to caring for a person suffering from dementia.

When should families consider a nursing home for a person with dementia? Many families agonize over this decision – when to seek an appropriate nursing home for the person. Husbands, wives, or adult children who have worked to keep the person suffering from dementia at home may feel a sense of failure and guilt when they begin to consider nursing home placement. Each family's ability to maintain the person at home is different due to many factors: the level of functioning varies from person to person; the availability of community resources differs widely; and the health and energy levels of family members to provide care will vary. Because of all these factors, no fixed guidelines can dictate when a person with a diagnosis of dementia needs nursing home care.

Safety

One important factor to consider is the person's safety. When staying at one's home without supervision is dangerous, alternatives should be considered. If a person lives alone and begins to forget to turn off the gas on the stove, the person's safety and well-being must be considered. The health of the caregiver also affects decisions about keeping a person suffering from dementia at home. If the demands of caregiving begin to jeopardize or compromise the caregiver's health, other options must be considered in order to obtain a balance that considers the person with a diagnosis of dementia and the caregiver. (NW, 2010)

Decisions Which Must be Made in Caring for
Individuals with a Diagnosis of Dementia

Relocation: when will it be necessary and where to relocate (such as a relative's home, Assisted Living facility, or Nursing Home)

Driving: When to limit or stop driving? How to accomplish this? Who will accomplish this? And who will be the driver and caregiver for the individual who is no longer driving?

Financial & Legal issues: Costs of care and living arrangements, resources to afford care, and who will be the decision-maker in regards to care of the individual with a diagnosis of dementia – Both financial and medical decision-making

Daily care: Who will assist with daily care including bathing, grooming, eating, toileting, and other household activities? Who will manage finances and daily expenses of living? Who will make the decisions regarding healthcare?

End-of-life care: Who will make decisions regarding continuity of care and decisions at the end of life?

In most families, there is generally one individual who will be the person who assumes the role of primary caregiver and decision-maker, but there are always others who are involved in making the decisions regarding an individual's care. There can be conflicts and disagreements about care when emotions are involved. There are other issues to consider: there is lack of understanding regarding the dementing disease; an inability to accept the deterioration of an individual's abilities and cognitive status; dysfunctional family relationships; or a combination of these factors.

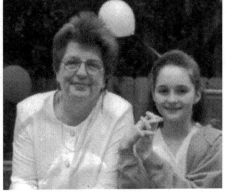

228

Problems Where Family Conflict Can Arise

What is the problem?

Whose problem is it?

Who's to decide?

What's to do?

Who's to do it?

When to do it?

Where to do it?

How to do it?

Family Conflict

Family members may disagree about care choices for their loved one who has a diagnosis of dementia. They may argue amongst themselves, they may neglect the problems that are obvious, they may blame others for their loved one's behaviors or their loved one's decline, or they may attempt to change many of the decisions which have already been made. Any, or all, of these behaviors of family members can occur, which can lead to conflict between family members or families and healthcare providers.

In order to manage conflict within a family, there are certain steps which will assist in creating a solution. Begin by discovering the family's problem; is the problem: a lack of knowledge regarding the disease or the person's declining abilities; role conflict among family members; inability to afford care for the person with a diagnosis of dementia; or another issue. The key to resolving family conflict is to define the problem and learn the meaning of the problem as identified by the family members involved.

It may help to investigate previous methods of intervention which family members have used in the past to resolve conflict. Next, identify and organize resources which may be available both within the family and from outside resources.

229

Managing Family Conflict: Ways to Intervene

Communication

Crisis intervention

Problem solving

Education

Social support

Conflict resolution

Family therapies

Suggestions for Families in Managing Care of an Individual with a Diagnosis of Dementia

Share responsibility: Ideally, family members should share the responsibility in care. In some cases, this does not occur. Caregivers should consider each family member's preferences, resources and abilities - physical, mental, and financial. Some family members may be able to provide hands-on care, either in their own homes or in the individual's home. Others may be more comfortable with offering financial assistance for care, assisting with household chores, or running errands for the caregiver. Others may be better suited to handling financial or legal issues.

Talking regularly or Meeting regularly can assist families in caring for an individual suffering with dementia. If there are issues a family is unable to discuss, family conflict is present, or additional resources are necessary – counselors or other family conflict management sources may be needed. It is encouraging to plan regular face-to-face family meetings. It is advisable to include everyone who's part of the family and the caregiving team, including family, friends, and other close contacts. Discuss each person's caregiving responsibilities and challenges in order to make changes accordingly. If time, distance or other logistical problems are issues for certain family members, consider conference calls, share email updates with the entire family, or start a family blog. If family meetings tend to turn into arguments, consider asking a counselor, social worker or other professional to moderate.

Be honest and talk about feelings in an open, constructive manner to help defuse tension. If certain family members are feeling stressed or overwhelmed, they should be encouraged to let others know – then they can work together to brainstorm about more effective ways to share the burden of care. A family should be careful to express feelings without blaming or shaming anyone else. Avoid using 'I' statements, such as 'I'm having trouble juggling my own schedule with all of Dad's appointments.' Keep an open mind while listening to other family members share their thoughts and feelings.

Don't criticize, since there are many 'right' ways to provide care. Respect each caregiver's abilities, style and values. Be especially supportive of family members responsible for daily, hands-on care since this can be a difficult and sometimes thankless task.

Consider counseling if there is concern that the stress of a person's dementia will tear the family apart, remind family members to seek help when the pressures of the disease, care, and life in general become too much. Families should be encouraged to consider joining a support group for Alzheimer's caregivers or seeking family counseling. Remember, working through conflicts together can help move families on to more important things like caring for an individual with dementia and enjoying this time together as much as possible.

(MayoClinic, 2010)

Chapter 9 References

HealthCentral.com (2010). Family Caregivers Often Delay Seeking Assistance Until Crisis Points. Retrieved July 10, 2010 from http://www.healthcentral.com/alzheimers/news-25914-5.html

MayoClinic (2010). Alzheimer's: Dealing with family conflict. Retrieved July 10, 2010 from http://health.msn.com/health-topics/caregiving/articlepage.aspx?cp-documentid=100096541

NW (2010). Family Caregiver Issues. Retrieved July 10, 2010 from http://www.brain.northwestern.edu/patients/family.html

Chapter 10

Caregivers of individuals with dementia often experience depression, anxiety, loneliness, isolation, and self-neglect. These issues can lead to stress and burn-out, even resulting in the caregiver dying before the one for whom they provide care. This chapter will present the signs and symptoms of caregiver stress and burnout as well as ways to manage and survival tips.

Introduction

The issues involved in caring for individuals with dementia often leave a person speechless. There are a multitude of issues and potentially difficult situations which occur that are not easy to manage – from loss of driving to loss of independence and eventually final dependence on another person for all aspects of living. Caregiving is stressful because it can drain a person physically as well as emotionally. Caregivers are not just dealing with objects such as the car, clothing, or food. Caregivers are providing care for human beings who are each unique individuals. These human beings are more than physical bodies – they come with a past, have lived their lives and should be respected for who they are as well as who they once were. And it must be remembered that they still have minds and spirits. This means that, in addition to doing the physical caregiving tasks, caregivers must also focus on the person by showing concern, listening, offering support, looking out for the person's best interest, and being compassionate and caring. This must be done when the caregiver may be tired and may not have enough emotional reserve to keep going.

- What does an adult child say to her Mom when she's run into the mailbox for the 4th time?
- How does a son ask his Dad if he's taking his medications like he should?

- How do siblings approach their parents about needing more help around the house?
- How do you tell an independent parent it's time to stop driving?

These issues can be challenging even in the closest of families where everyone is cooperating and working for the good of the individual with a diagnosis of dementia and the family as a whole. But there may be conflicts within families, differing opinions or understanding of the person's cognitive abilities and level of functioning, or the person suffering from dementia continues in the disease progression and not everyone believes the person is worsening (and that happens). It is sometimes easier not to admit there is a problem or not to talk at all, which can lead to unresolved issues. The fact is that many times, the problem is not recognized because children are caught up in the day-to-day hectic schedules of their own families and awareness of the issues arising in an aging relative are not discovered until a catastrophic event occurs, such as a fall and an accident.

Talking sooner is better than later or waiting until a crisis, which can lead to conflict and disagreements in care and may not be in the person with dementia's best interest (Senior Care, 2010). Admitting there are changes in a person is the first step to diagnosis and appropriate care. When a diagnosis of dementia is suspected or confirmed, now the journey begins.

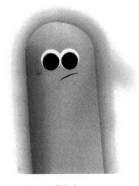

A Senior Moment or Something Else

Early on, I had my suspicions but still could convince myself she was just getting older and there wasn't really anything major to worry about. She was a little forgetful, but as Mom told me 'I'm just like everyone my age, we all forget things a little.' One day, I stopped by Mom's house after work, as I often did to see how she was doing and to bring her the items from the store she had called and asked me to pick up. Upon entering the house, Mom said, 'Well I wish you had called, I needed something from the store.' I reminded her that I had spoken to her earlier and had been instructed to bring these items from the store by her house after work. She looked puzzled, insisting she had not spoken to me that day, even arguing with me about it. This made me realize, maybe there was something more to the issue and there was a problem which needed attention. I discussed the issue with my sister, who initially didn't want to believe there was a 'big' problem but believed me and agreed this was something to be investigated further. I discussed my concerns with Mom who did not want to admit anything was wrong but agreed to have a medical work-up. Thankfully, we could talk about the problem, both with Mom as well as my sister, and we worked together to get an accurate diagnosis and treatment plan. Now I will say, this did not occur overnight; initially my sister wanted to deny there was a problem, as well as Mom refusing to believe there was a problem, but there were small things that kept adding to the bigger picture – there was a list of problems: sleeping all day and up all night, forgetting she had gone to the store and purchased certain items and making an additional trip for the same item. It was just a multitude of small things and, when looking back, I realized that I should have recognized the problem earlier than later.

Is Mom Safe at Home

Living in one's own home and being self-sufficient means independence. It can also be a major factor affecting an individual's self-esteem. When adult individuals who are very independent and have lived, worked, and raised their own families are no longer able to care for themselves without assistance, a person's freedom and independence may be in jeopardy of being taken away. The major issues involved in making decisions which restrict a person's freedom revolve around safety and well-being. When risks are great enough to outweigh a person's wish to remain independent, alternative solutions may be necessary. But how does a caregiver determine when a person should no longer be driving? When a person can no longer (safely) be independent? And what does it mean when you take away that person's independence by either having them move to live with someone else or move to an Assisted Living Facility or a Nursing Home? What will that person do when he/she needs to go somewhere or needs something? Taking away a person's independence can in essence create a dependent person. And upon whom will that person depend? Often it is the person who takes measures to safeguard the person, who takes away a person's independence, who is now the 'caregiver'. Thus it is often easier to ignore the problem. But those individuals who make the choice to help a person with dementia should be supported because it is not an easy task and is often a thankless and tiring one as well (Senior Care, 2010). After identifying that a person should no longer live independently, next the caregiver must assess how much independence is necessary to restrict and how quickly to impose these restrictions. Some individuals function well during the daytime but become confused in the evening and night-time hours. Some individuals require care on a 24-hour-a-day basis. This will vary from person to person and from situation to situation.

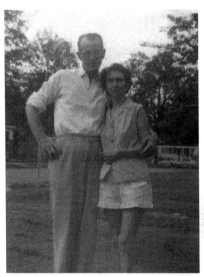

Caregiver

A caregiver is anyone who provides care, helps another person, and has the responsibility for another person, often 24 hours a day, seven days a week. Initially, many individuals with cognitive impairment may be able to live independently and only need assistance in paying bills, grocery shopping, and driving. But as a person's dementia progresses, the person may become more and more dependent for even their most basic needs. Caring for individuals suffering from dementia may mean providing care to someone who has a condition which requires assistance with all activities of daily living such as eating, bathing, and toileting. But many times making sure a person's basic needs are satisfied can be difficult when the caregiver is met with resistance from the person needing care due behavioral problems, as well as psychiatric issues such as anxiety, depression, confusion, disorientation, cognitive impairment, and other behavioral problems. Caregivers have many duties including helping the ill person with:

- grocery shopping
- house cleaning
- laundry

- cooking
- shopping
- paying bills
- taking medicine
- bathing
- using the toilet
- dressing
- eating
- getting to bed

People who are not paid to provide care are known as informal caregivers and are often family members. Other types of caregiver relationships include:

- adults caring for other relatives – including grandparents, siblings, aunts, and uncles
- spouses caring for elderly husbands or wives
- middle-aged parents caring for severely disabled adult children
- adults caring for friends and neighbors
- children caring for a disabled parent or elderly grandparent

Most people will be informal caregivers at some point during their lives. During any given year, there are more than 44 million Americans – that's 21% of the adult population – who provide unpaid care to an elderly person. Informal caregivers provide 80% of care on a long-term basis in the United States: 61% of caregivers are women, most caregivers are middle-aged, and 13% of caregivers are aged 65 years and older. Over half of informal caregivers have jobs in addition to caring for another person. Because of time spent caregiving, more than half of employed female caregivers must make changes at work, including going in late, leaving early, missing work, or working fewer hours (HHS, 2010).

Rewards of Caregiving

Although caregiving can be challenging, it is important to note that it can also have its rewards:

❖ Feelings of giving back to a loved one or another person
❖ Stronger relationship with loved one or another person
❖ Learning to appreciate life more
❖ Feeling good about self

But caregiver stress can occur. Caregiver stress appears to affect women more than men because women are more often the caregiver. About 75% of caregivers report feeling very strained emotionally, physically, and/or financially.

(HHS, 2010)

Caregiver Stress

Caregiver stress is the emotional and physical stress caused by the strain of providing care to another person. A recent study demonstrated that 76% of family caregivers reported their aging loved one's needs to be overwhelming, 91% said they have episodes of anxiety or irritable, 73% have disturbed sleep patterns and 56% seem to become ill more frequently (Senior Care, 2010). Caregiver stress can take many forms.

Symptoms of Caregiver Stress

• Frustration and anger that may result from from taking care of someone with dementia who often wanders away or becomes easily upset
• Guilt because many think that they should be able to provide better care, despite all the other things that they have to do
• Loneliness because all the time spent caregiving has hurt the caregiver's social life
• Exhaustion

Caregiver Stress Effects on Health

Caring for another person can be extremely difficult, especially with an individual who has not only physical needs but also psychiatric issues and behavioral problems. All of these issues combined are physically demanding as well as emotionally draining.

Caregiver Stress and Burnout

It can affect the mental and physical health of a caregiver. Some caregivers are in good health but some have serious health problems themselves. Research shows that caregivers:

- are more likely to be have symptoms of depression or anxiety
- are more likely to have a long-term medical problem, such as heart disease, cancer, diabetes, or arthritis
- have higher levels of stress hormones
- spend more days sick with an infectious disease
- have a weaker immune response to the influenza, or flu, vaccine
- have slower wound healing
- have higher levels of obesity
- may be at higher risk for mental decline, including problems with memory and paying attention

(HHS, 2010)

*One research study found that older caregivers who felt stressed while taking care of their disabled spouses were 63% more likely to die within 4 years than caregivers who were not feeling stressed. This is concerning because after the caregiver has died, the person for whom they were caring may no longer have anyone to help them and may require placement in a Nursing Home or other facility.

Caregiver issues which contribute to this problem include personal health problems that are exacerbated when individuals do not take good care of themselves. Many caregivers, as compared to individuals who are not caregivers, are less likely to:

- get necessary medical care
- take medications as prescribed
- seek preventive care such as mammograms, routine pap smears, or prostate exams
- exercise regularly
- eat nutritiously
- get an adequate amount of sleep

Identifying Caregiver Stress

Being a Caregiver may place a great deal of stress on an individual. Symptoms of Caregiver Stress include:

- feeling overwhelmed
- sleeping problems, either too much or too little
- changes in weight, either gaining or losing
- fatigue – feeling tired most of the time
- loss of interest in activities which were pleasurable
- becoming easily irritated or angered
- feeling constantly worried
- depression or often feeling sad
- anxiety
- chronic discomfort, for example frequent headaches, bodily pain, or other physical problems
- abuse of alcohol or drugs, including prescription drugs

Preventing Burnout and Relieving Stress

Caregiver stress can lead to serious health problems and 'burnout'. Burnout isn't like a cold. It is not always easily noticed and may not become apparent until it escalates into a full-blown depression or burnout. Very much like Post Traumatic Stress Syndrome, the symptoms of burnout can surface over months to years. Symptoms of burnout in an individual might not be noticed by a person but others might say they see the symptoms of anxiety, depression, or burnout in a caregiver. Think about what is being said about a caregiver and consider the possibility of burnout (Seligson, 2010). Steps should be taken to reduce stress as much as possible. Research shows that people who take an active, problem-solving approach to caregiving issues are less likely to feel stressed than those who react by worrying and feeling helpless. Some facilities and church groups offer classes that can teach caregivers how to care for someone with dementia. There are also support groups whose members can share creative ways to manage problems. To find these classes, ask a healthcare provider, contact an organization that focuses on this disease, or call the local Area Agency on Aging. Other good sources of caregiving information include:

- healthcare providers
- library books
- web sites of disease-specific organizations

More Tips for Reducing Caregiver Stress

- Try to find time to be physically active on a routine basis, eat a healthy diet, and get enough sleep.
- Find out about caregiving resources in the community.
- Ask for and accept help! AND be prepared with a mental list of ways that others can help and let the helper choose what they can do; for example, one person might be happy to take the person with dementia on a walk a couple times a week. Someone else might be glad to pick up some groceries.
- If you, as a caregiver, need financial help taking care of a relative, don't be afraid to ask family members to contribute their fair share. BE CONCRETE: Do not expect family members to know when financial help is needed – ask for X amount of money every month; Do not expect helpers to know when to come by to help; ask helpers for specific assistance, such as someone to come for 2 hours every other Saturday – BE SPECIFIC!
- Say 'No' to requests that are draining, such as hosting holiday meals.
- Don't feel guilty that you are not a 'perfect' caregiver. Just as there is no 'perfect parent', there is no such thing as a 'perfect caregiver'. Caregivers are doing the best they can.
- Identify what you, as a caregiver, can and cannot change: The caregiver may not be able to change someone else's behavior, but can change the way that he/she reacts to the person exhibiting problematic behaviors
- Set realistic goals. Break large tasks into smaller steps that can done one at a time.

- Prioritize, make lists, and establish a daily routine.
- Stay in touch with family and friends.
- Join a support group for caregivers in the same situation, such as caring for someone with dementia. Besides being a great way to make new friends, caregivers can also pick up some caregiving tips from others who are facing the same problems.
- Make time each week to do something that the caregiver wants to do, such as going to see a movie.
- See healthcare providers for a checkup. Tell them that you are a caregiver and mention any symptoms of depression or sickness.
- Try to keep a sense of humor.
- As a caregiver, pat yourself on the back for everything you are doing.

If working outside the home and feeling overwhelmed, a caregiver should consider taking a break from their job. Employees covered under the Federal Family and Medical Leave Act may be able to take unpaid leave to care for relatives.

Caregiving Services in the Community

There are many programs and services, nationally as well as locally, which can provide help for caregivers.
- transportation
- meal delivery
- home health care services such as nursing or physical therapy
- non-medical home care services such as housekeeping, cooking, or companionship
- home modification such as changes to the home that make it easier for a person suffering from dementia to perform basic daily tasks, such as bathing, using the toilet, and moving around
- legal and financial counseling

When Caregivers Need a Break

Taking some time off from caregiving can reduce stress. 'Respite care' provides substitute caregiving to allow the regular caregiver a much-needed break. Below are the various types of respite services that are available:

- In-home respite: A type of service where someone comes to the home of a person to provide care, ranging from simple companionship to nursing services.
- Adult day-care centers: Many adult day-care centers are located in churches or community centers. Some day-care centers provide care for older adults similar to care provided by child day-care centers but geared to meet the needs of the older person as well as provide an outlet for socialization.
- Short-term nursing homes. If the caregiver needs occasional nursing care or must leave town for a couple weeks; some nursing homes will offer short-term placement.

Devices that can Help Provide Care

There are devices that can be purchased that can help make sure that a person with dementia is safe.

- **Emergency response systems** involve a button on a necklace, bracelet, or belt that the person with dementia wears. If there is an emergency and the caregiver is not home, the person presses the button to alert a monitoring center. The center then alerts medical personnel and the caregiver. These systems are intended for people who can press the button and do not have dementia, or who are in the earlier stages of dementia.
- An **intercom system** allows caregivers to hear a person with dementia from another area of the home.
- A **Webcam** is a video camera that allows the caregiver to see a person with dementia from another area of the home.
- **Mobility monitors** use a small transmitter to help keep track of individuals with dementia. When a person suffering from

dementia wearing a transmitter strapped to their ankle or wrist passes outside of a set range, the transmitter alerts the caregiver that the person with dementia is wandering away.

Also, researchers are developing technologies to allow healthcare providers to examine and treat individuals from locations different than the healthcare provider's office. This new field is called telemedicine. It uses a communication system, like the Internet or two-way television, to collect medical information and provide instructions to the caregiver and patient. Telemedicine will be most useful in rural areas where few healthcare providers are available. Some states already have limited telemedicine programs in operation.

Finding Caregiving Services in the Local Community

The Area Agency on Aging (AAA) can provide information on local services and allows caregivers to learn about services where they live. AAA is usually listed in the city or county government sections of the telephone directory under "Aging" or "Health and Human Services." The National Eldercare Locator is another service of the U.S. Administration on Aging which can also help caregivers in their local AAA.

Paying for Home Health Care and Other Caregiving Services

Medicare, Medicaid, and private insurance companies will cover some of the costs of home health care and services. Some costs may be covered by payer plans but others may not and will have to be paid for directly by an individual.

The cost of home care depends upon what services are needed. Services generally covered by insurance include: an individual with dementia having unstable medical problems that require monitoring or stabilization or a caregiver needs to be taught a skill to care for the person with dementia. Non-covered expenses may include:

housecleaning duties, bathing and grooming assistance. In certain states, insurance plans may provide coverage for modifying a home so the individual will be safer and be able to 'age in place,' i.e., stay in their own home as long as possible.

To find out if what is covered and which individuals are eligible for Medicare home health care services, read the free publication *Medicare and Home Health Care* (Publication No. CMS-10969) available on the internet at http://www.medicare.gov/Publications/Pubs/pdf/10969.pdf. Caregivers can also call with their Regional Home Health Intermediary. To locate the phone number, on the internet – search Contacts Database of the Centers for Medicare & Medicaid Services at: http://www.cms.hhs.gov/apps/contacts. Or call 1-800-MEDICARE (1-800-633-4227).

To qualify for Medicaid, an individual must have a low income and few other assets. To find out if a person qualifies for Medicaid, call the State Medical Assistance Office. To find the phone number, go to the Contacts Database of the Centers for Medicare & Medicaid Services at: http://www.cms.hhs.gov/apps/contacts.

Besides Medicare and Medicaid, there is another federal program, called the National Family Caregiver Support Program, that helps states provide services for family caregivers. To be eligible for the program, a caregiver must meet certain criteria:

- providing care for an adult aged 60 years and older
- caring for a person of any age with Alzheimer's disease or a related disorder
- be a grandparent or relative 55 years of age or older who is the primary caregiver of a child under the age of 18
- be a grandparent or relative 55 years of age or older providing care to an adult, aged 18 to 59 years with a disability

Each state offers different amounts and types of services. These include:

- information about available services
- help accessing support services
- individual counseling and organization of support groups

- caregiver training
- respite care
- supplemental services, supplies, and equipment, such as home modifications, emergency response systems, nutritional supplements, incontinence supplies, etc.

To access services under the National Family Caregiver Support Program, contact the local Area Agency on Aging.

— — — — — — — — — — — — — —

Caregivers who have actively lived their lives, been involved with others, and attempted to walk on unfamiliar paths, have probably made a fair share of mistakes.

Although making mistakes can be a difficult – even painful – experience to go through, mistakes also offer a rich opportunity for growth. They provide insights that people would otherwise not know. They also offer lessons about patience and forgiveness.

Although no one wants to make mistakes, they are important life lessons for people.

(AALTCN-Affirmations, 2010)

Chapter 10 References

AALTCN. (2010). Affirmations. Retrieved May 3, 2010.

HHS. (2010). Caregiver Stress. Retrieved April 18, 2010 from
http://www.womenshealth.gov/FAQ/caregiver-stress.cfm

Senior Care. (2010). Running on Empty. Retrieved on April
21, 2010 from http://www.homeinstead.com/resources/
familyresources/Running%20on%20Empty.aspx

Seligson, M. (2010). Caregiver Burnout. Retrieved August, 1,
2010 from http://www.caregiver.com/articles/caregiver/
caregiver_burnout.htm

Chapter 11

Ethics of Care

Alzheimer's disease and other dementias have a physiological cause, are progressive disorders, and are terminal diseases. Individuals who have these diseases often are not rational and many times are not allowed to choose the direction of their care – someone else makes the decisions for them because they often cannot think clearly and logically. There are many ethical issues to consider and this chapter discusses some of the issues surrounding truth telling and autonomy of cognitively impaired individuals. There will also be a brief discussion about justice – offering similar care to all no matter their financial status, race, religion, or cognitive ability.

Introduction

Imagine, the feelings of fear, rejection, frustration, shame, and reluctance that surge through a caregiver when they realize a person cannot toilet themselves without help any longer...

Imagine, the grieving a caregiver experiences as the hope that it isn't really Alzheimer's is dashed, and there is a definitive diagnosis that a person has a progressive, terminal illness and there will be total dependence for all activities such as eating, bathing, & toileting until the person dies...

Imagine, the effort it takes to live, hide the fears, ignore the stigmatization and inherent taboos, the grieving and the acknowledgment that the situation will not improve, as they go on day-by-day and find ways to cope with the situation...

Now **Imagine** being the person who is suffering from dementia and this is all about you.

A True Story: Mom had always had a bit of a problem with constipation but things had seemed to have gotten worse. Mom was in the early stages of Alzheimer's disease but we did not know yet (for sure). She was still independent, but you could tell she had a few memory problems. One day, she started vomiting while at the store shopping and complained of constipation. It was bad enough for me to take her to a local Emergency Room. She was briefly examined and diagnosed with constipation, given a laxative and sent home. The problem did not get any better and after 3 more days, we returned to the Emergency Room (no bowel movement yet). She was again examined, diagnosed with constipation and given a laxative, sent home. 3 days later, we were back at the Emergency Room, same story, diagnosed with constipation, told to take a laxative, and she was about to be discharged again. I (as a Nurse myself) said NO! There was something more wrong and we needed further evaluation. At my insistence, she was admitted. They did X-Rays and exams as well as blood work. They gave her multiple laxatives (some really powerful ones too), about 5 a day, as well as other therapies. She did not eat since she was vomiting also and she was given fluids through an Intravenous Infusion (IV).

After 5 days, I finally caught up with her doctor and was told that 'this was the worst case of constipation I have ever seen' – to my amazement (I think my mouth dropped and stayed open). I finally decided enough was enough, I made arrangements to have Mom taken somewhere else for further evaluation and was about to leave 'against medical advice' when I told her nurse as well as physician that this was neglect – if not worse – the M word (Malpractice). Well this really got everyone's attention. That night, she had a CT scan done of her abdomen and was on the operating table the next morning. We received a diagnosis of Colon cancer which had already extensively metastasized so it was pretty advanced. The main issue was that her complaints were not taken as seriously as those of someone who was cognitively intact. This was not right or fair ... but it happened.

The society in which we live often views individuals who are suffering from dementia as less than... And once an individual receives a diagnosis of dementia, things change. Sometimes these individuals may have difficulty in verbalizing what they think, feel, or wish. Sometimes they cannot interpret the things their bodies are telling them such as constipation or the need to urinate. Sometimes they are no longer listened to in the same way and sometimes their complaints are not taken seriously. Sometimes they are overlooked or ignored. Society has a tendency to stigmatize these individuals and not offer or provide the same choices, the same care, or the same opportunities as those provided to individuals who do not have a diagnosis of dementia. This is one of the reasons many people do not want to know they have a dementia, including Alzheimer's disease. If they did know and accepted that diagnosis, they would be admitting they were destined to lose their ability to think and make decisions, their ability to be independent – to go where they want to and when they want to, and they would be viewed as less than...

251

Values and Guiding Principles

Ethics guides life and all healthcare professionals' practices. There are some guiding principles which should be embedded in the way anyone thinks about and acts around individuals with dementia.

Respect: Show respect for the dignity of the person suffering from dementia

Compassion: Show concern and understanding, and support the personhood of individuals suffering from dementia

Integrity: Focus on trustworthiness, including honesty, reliability and loyalty, in an environment of total all-encompassing care

Competency: Focus on effective, appropriate, high-quality care and administration in programs and services for people suffering from dementia and their families

Justice: Offer the same care to all individuals and do not be prejudiced due to race, sex, religion, financial status, or cognitive abilities

Beneficence: Do 'Good' for the person!

Nonmalificence: Do no 'harm'!

Guiding Principles

Many types of dementia, including Alzheimer's disease are progressive, degenerative diseases of the brain that have profound impacts on people with the disease and their families. People suffering from dementia should be told about their diagnosis and made aware of available treatment options; must have access to current information, and receive appropriate coordinated care as well as support from knowledgeable, healthcare professionals. These individuals need to participate in decision-making regarding their daily lives and future care for as long as they are able. If unable to participate, a surrogate decision maker may need to assist with making choices but the known values and wishes of the person should be used to guide all decisions. People with dementia need a safe, restraint-free living environment, and protection from neglect, exploitation and/or abuse. Family and friends who care for people suffering from dementia need to have their caregiving needs assessed and provided for. All involved, both the individuals with dementia and those who care for them need to take an active role in the planning and implementation of care. Adequate resources should be available to provide support to people with dementia and their caregivers throughout the course of the person's life and their illness.

Living

An increasing number of older individuals are living alone. If they also have a diagnosis of Alzheimer's disease or another dementia, they are more likely to be diagnosed later in the disease because their symptoms often go unrecognized. Our society values independence and the ability to be independent. Moving people away from their homes to live with someone else or into a Nursing Home type of setting, is often viewed as a loss of independence. This is not necessarily so, as a move may offer people not only support and safety but also an environment that encourages independence and offers socialization.

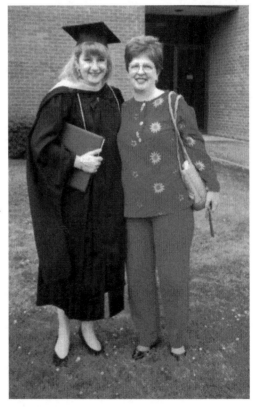

The Issues

Premature move from home: The person with a diagnosis of dementia may have a higher tolerance for risk than others (family members and caregivers) and may receive pressure to move out of their home earlier than necessary.

Determining when living alone is no longer safe or desirable: For people who no longer have an understanding of their own safety and ability to look after themselves, others often have to determine if it is still suitable for the person to live alone. The risks of living alone must be weighed against the benefits of providing the care and support that enables the person to live at home.

Barriers within the health-care, community care and legal systems: Caregivers often face barriers when trying to determine if a move from home is needed or if additional support can assist in keeping a person in their own home. These barriers include the difficulty of sharing information due to privacy and confidentiality regulations; the limited availability of services to support independent living as well as the high costs; and the complexities of competency legislation i.e., the laws that determine when a person is no longer able to make a certain decision.

Loss of independence: Some individuals who have a diagnosis of dementia realize when living alone is no longer safe or desirable. Others may want to stay in their own home for as long as possible, even if there are some safety issues – since moving away from home may be viewed as a loss of self-reliance and control in their daily lives. But, the problem is that some individuals do not realize when living alone is no longer safe and this is the problem.

(Alzheimer's Society, 2010)

Living Environments that Provide Safety, Quality of Life and Support

People with dementia should live in environments that best support their safety, health, and quality of life. For some, this may mean living at home with support services, even if there is some risk. If problems have been identified, it is important that caregivers try to lessen them, wherever possible.

- If a person frequently leaves the stove on, consider disconnecting the stove
- If a person wanders outside and could become lost, consider taking walks with the person or providing a safe environment in which the person may walk
- If a person is unable to cook for him/herself, find other ways to provide hot food – Meals-on-Wheels programs, have a friend or neighbor drop by at mealtimes, or have pre-made meals available, etc.

The amount and type of support available are important factors in determining if a person can stay independent and continue to live alone. A person with a large family living in a community with many services may be better able to live alone than someone with no family living in a community with limited or no services. Wherever possible, the person suffering from dementia should take part in discussions concerning whether or not to continue living alone.

Some Factors to Consider

Overall well-being

- Is the person physically able to live independently?
- Does the person have a good quality of life at home?
- Is there enough stimulation during the day?
- Could the person benefit from the level of care and support provided by another environment such as with a relative or friend, Assisted Living Facility or Nursing Home?

Ethics of Care

Health

- Is the person able to take medication properly?
- Has the person had any problems with falling?
- If sick, would the person be able to understand and take appropriate action, such as calling for help?
- Is the person able to take care of daily activities such as personal hygiene, bathing and toileting?
- Are there current or past health problems that might put the person at risk of harm?

Nutrition

- Has the person had any changes in weight?
- Is the person able to eat nutritiously throughout the day?
- Is the person able to store foods properly?
- Can the person prepare the foods safely?

Safety

- Is the person at risk of harm? If yes, is the amount of risk acceptable to all involved (the person, family members, and other caregivers)?
- Does the person pose a risk to self or others? For example, does the person smoke cigarettes and fall asleep – which could cause fires? Or does the person forget they are cooking and could cause a fire with the stove?
- Is the person able to react and take action in an emergency, such as a fire?
- Is the person's home safe? For example, are stairs well lit? Are there handrails?

Finances

- Can the person handle day-to-day financial transactions, such as paying bills?
- Is the person at risk of exploitation or abuse regarding finances?

Strategies to Enhance Independent Living

The following strategies may help provide support to a person with dementia who lives alone.

Safety	**Keep a set of house keys with trusted family member or neighbors & Arrange for someone to call or visit once a day**
	Appliance safety measures: Automatic shut off kettle Stove safety – remove fuses, put burners on timers, shut off gas Lower temperature of hot water heater
	Emergency call system so there is 24-hour access to help should a problem arise
Daily living	Get the person assistance with tasks, such as housekeeping and meal preparation
	Assist in sorting closets and dresser drawers to make only the necessary clothes available
Food	Arrange Meals-on-Wheels for hot food delivery
	Provide a toaster oven or microwave for heating food
	Use prepared foods, non-perishable foods and foods that do not need to be stored in a refrigerator
Medication	Simplify medication routines – use a pill dispenser or have someone visit to give pills
	Use a calendar for the person to document that he/she has taken morning & evening pills
	Only allow access to a small number of pills over a specified period of time
Finances	Bank-at-home services
	Make someone else, such as a substitute decision-maker, responsible for handling finances such as writing checks, paying bills, monitoring accounts
	Direct deposit of checks and direct payment of bills

Living in a place that is safe, familiar and comfortable is important to everyone, including individuals suffering from dementia. Some individuals may be capable of living on their own for some time after a diagnosis of dementia. Others may be at too much risk to continue living alone. It is often difficult to decide when living at home is puts the person at too much risk. However, it is better to allow an individual to continue to stay in their routine, at their homes for as long as possible, and avoid a premature move from home. Each person's living situation should be monitored and assessed carefully, as the disease progresses.

Decision-making: Respecting Individual Choice

Making decisions and controlling one's own life are important for each of us. It is no different for the person suffering from dementia. However, the extent to which a confused person can make simple or complex decisions varies greatly and the ability to allow a confused individual to make decisions will be dependent on the gravity of the decision as well as the consequences of the choice. **Opportunities to make decisions**: As a person's dementia progresses, decision-making abilities will change and caregivers may choose to make all decisions and not present these individuals with a diagnosis of dementia with opportunities to make decisions of their own. This may occur not just with simple day-to-day decisions but also decisions relating to a person's future care and support. **Respect for the person's wishes**: Respect how a person would have wanted their care directed, when they could have made a rationale choice. Sometimes those making decisions on behalf of the person with the disease do not use the person's wishes as a guide and put their own interests first.

Substitute Decision-makers and Health-care Professionals

Assessment of abilities: Determine a person's cognitive reasoning abilities and the impact of the decision. Caregivers may find it difficult to confront the person about the loss of decision-making abilities and may choose not to take action even though they know that the person is making poor decisions.

Decision-making strategies: Be aware of strategies that help make it easier for people with dementia to make many of their own decisions. Or perhaps caregivers may not realize how important decision-making can be to maintaining a person's confidence and self-esteem.

Challenges of substitute decision-making: As a person loses decision-making capabilities, decision-making will involve others. It can be difficult and highly stressful to make decisions on behalf of another person. This is particularly so when the values and wishes of the person with dementia are unknown, unclear or impossible to follow. Also, the wishes of the ill person may conflict with those of the substitute decision-maker, family or society. Also, if several family members are involved in making decisions, they may not be able to agree upon what the ill person's wishes are.

Preferred choices

- **Recognize abilities**
  Recognize that the person still has abilities. These abilities should be respected and encouraged. Support a person in making decisions independently, and involve the person in decision-making while capable. Create a plan for the time to determine when a person will not be able to make independent decisions.

- **Plan for the future**
  While able, the person suffering from dementia and the substitute decision-maker should take the opportunity to discuss openly and frankly issues relating to future health care, personal care and financial decisions. Wherever possible, legal paperwork should be completed to ensure that the wishes of the person are recognized as well as recorded and a substitute decision-maker is named. Check with local regulations regarding requirements.

- **Adjust to changing abilities**
  As the disease progresses and the person's abilities decline, those involved in care should identify what abilities the person still has, break down complex tasks and decisions into more easily-managed options, and respect the person's choices. Remember, there will be cognitive decline over time and what a person can do this year, may change next year.
- **Respect a person's values and wishes**
  When the time comes that a person is unable to make decisions, the substitute decision-maker should follow the expressed wishes of that person. When these wishes are not known, the substitute decision-maker should make the decision based on what is thought the person would want. The risks of a decision must be weighed against the benefits of any decision, and the decision-maker should assess how it will affect the person's quality of life and well-being. Allow as much decision making as possible, for as long as possible.

Strategies to Facilitate Decision-making

- **Personal involvement**
  Feelings of independence and self-esteem are promoted when individuals are allowed some degree of control in the day-to-day details of life. As the abilities of a person suffering from dementia change, those providing care and supporting need to ensure that the person continues to be involved in making as many decisions as possible. Strategies to achieve this include:
  o Provide limited choices to encourage a person to choose, reduce the number of options at any one time. For example: Bad – open-ended questions such as 'what do you want to wear today?'; Good – limited choices such as 'would you like to wear the red dress or the green dress?'
  o Break down tasks and instructions – provide step-by-step guidance. For example: Bad – telling someone to do a task that has multiple steps: 'Brush your teeth'; Good – breaking

down tasks into singular steps: 'Let's brush our teeth, take the toothbrush and wet it please...'

○ Look, listen, & feel. Listen and be sensitive to messages that a person can convey by facial expression, tone of voice and body language. Feelings and emotions remain intact even after the ability to understand language has been lost.

- **Open discussion**

  Most people are not comfortable about making plans for a time when they will be unable to make decisions and will lose control of their own lives. Discussing personal values in relation to illness and death as well as finances and living arrangements are difficult. But avoiding the issues can result in people being denied the opportunity to express and realize their wishes about their own care.

  While they are still able to make decisions, people should be encouraged to discuss their choices and who their substitute decision-maker will be. Family members and substitute decisions-makers should be aware of what the person values and how the person defines quality of life. Discussion of these matters helps give the person a sense of control over their future decisions, and provides support and reassurance to the substitute decision-makers.

- **Substitute decision-making**

  Substitute decision-makers should be selected. It could be one person. Or, it could be one person for health-care decisions and another person for financial decisions. In choosing substitute decision-makers, consider their availability to take on the role, understanding and respect for the values and wishes of the person, ability to work with others, and ability to resolve conflicts.

- **Advance directive**

  The person's values and wishes should be written down in an advance directive. This is a document that records a person's wishes about their preferences in care. When a person becomes incapable of making decisions in the future, the advance directive will provide direction. It is also referred to by others terms, including living or enduring will or durable power of attorney for health care.

- **Competency assessment**

For some major decisions, it may be necessary to have experts assess the person's ability to make decisions.

- **When decisions become difficult**

If the time comes that a substitute decision-maker is called upon to make a decision on behalf of the person, the expressed wishes of the person should be followed whenever possible. If conflict develops, or, if the person's wishes are not known, are unclear or are impossible to follow, there should be a review of the decision based on:

○ the values of the person with dementia;
○ weighing the risks against the benefits of the decision;
○ the effect of the decision on the physical and emotional well-being of a person;
○ the effect of the decision on the quality of life of a person, caregivers and family members.

Disagreements may arise when there are differences in the needs and wishes of the individual and the caregivers; an impartial, trusted third party may need to be consulted to assist in resolving this type of issue. With some decisions, a resolution may take some time.

End-of-Life Decisions

Many dementias are terminal (can cause the death of the person). There are different approaches to treatment that need to be understood when making decisions for care in the later stage of this type of disease. Knowing in advance the person's wishes for these difficult situations can ease the burden of making decisions. However, some choices may not be appropriate if they would not improve the situation or may cause more harm than good.

Aggressive medical care is prolonging life using all available types of treatment.
This could happen in the hospital, a nursing home, or at the individual's home, such as using tube feeding when swallowing is no longer possible.

Conservative medical care is maintaining or attempting to improve current health status without using extremely aggressive measures. Care that is considered routine or usual practice, such as using blood pressure medication to treat high blood pressure, giving insulin for diabetes or antibiotics for an infection, or setting a fractured hip.

Comfort or palliative care is providing active and compassionate care when cure is not the goal. The priority is symptom management and pain control, as well as meeting the physical, emotional, spiritual, social and cultural needs of the person and the family.

(Alzheimer's Society, 2010)

Recognizing the cognitive abilities of the person suffering from dementia is the key to supporting decision-making that respects the person and offers opportunities to promote independence and self-esteem. When a person can no longer make decisions, the individual's values and wishes must be respected. These needs and wishes may have to be balanced with the needs and wishes of families, substitute decision-makers and health-care professionals. Keeping the balance is not always easy.

What can be done to enhance the quality of life of people suffering from dementia?
Individuals with dementia are still people and need to be treated with respect, integrity, compassion, and dignity. Those with mild to moderate symptoms may need to be supported by

finding opportunities to enhance their quality of life. As the disease progresses, preserving the quality of life of a person may require changing the environment to promote safety and meet the person's physical needs.

Some key elements to consider include:

- Learn about a person's dementia, understanding how it progresses, and knowing how to communicate with the person.
- Learn more about the person's particular likes, dislikes and opinions; or, if the person is unable to communicate this, talking to someone close to the person who knows the person can provide insight.
- Encourage independence and allow as much personal decision making as possible.
- Build on a person's strengths and abilities to encourage a sense of feeling useful.
- Ensure that the person's overall health is monitored and assessed, and that appropriate treatments are given.
- Provide a safe living environment which is also familiar for the person, while allowing a person to maintain remaining abilities.
- Respect a person's need for companionship, including physical intimacy. Relationships with family and friends should be fostered as much as possible.
- Provide care that responds to each person's needs and focuses on abilities rather than losses.
- Acknowledge and recognize that a person's interests may change over time.

Strategies to enhance the caregiver's quality of life include:

- Support:
  - Talk to close friends about your needs, the needs of the person being cared for and where the two sets of needs conflict.
  - Obtain support from groups or from one-on-one relationships.
- Take regular breaks from caregiving, for a few hours, days or weeks, and find activities that help you get away from caregiving responsibilities and tasks.
- Learn about signs of stress and develop ways to deal with them.
- Take satisfaction in the work you are doing to provide quality care.
- Learn to ask for help and accept it! Be specific: Ask for $X per month to help towards medication costs or ask someone to, "Come by and take Mom for a walk 3 days a week."
- Become aware of your own emotions, feelings, and reactions to stress. Take care of your needs throughout the course of the disease.
- Expect change: Plan for changes and recognize that there may be difficult decisions ahead.

(Alzheimer's Society, 2010; Alzheimer's for Caregivers, 2010)

Chapter 11 References

Alzheimer's for Caregivers. (2010). Bias and Alzheimer's disease. Retrieved April 21, 2010 from http://www.bigtreemurphy. com/Bias%20and%20Alzheimer's%20Disease.htm

Alzheimer's Society. (2010). Alzheimer's disease: Ethical Guidelines. Retrieved April 21, 2010 from http://www. alzheimer.ca/english/care/ethics-values.htm

Weiner, M. (2010). Legal and Ethical Issues for Patients with Dementia and Their Families. Geriatric Times. V (1). Retrieved April 21, 2010 from http://www.cmellc.com/ geriatrictimes/g040218.html

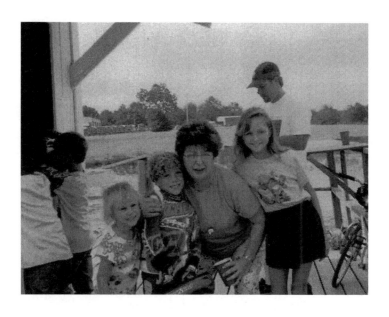

Chapter 12

Discussed in this chapter will be the legal issues which must be addressed in care of individuals with dementia, including assessing the decision-making ability of confused individuals, advanced directives, power-of-attorney – both medical and legal, guardianship, and important documents to locate. Also discussed will be the stages of dementia, common behaviors associated in the different stages, common triggers for behaviors, strategies to managing the problems AND SURVIVAL TIPS.

Introduction

Dementia is caused by a physiological disease and will progress and worsen over time. There are many causes of dementia but Alzheimer's disease (AD) is the most common cause of dementia in the older population. Some other dementias will progress through stages similar to those of AD. AD is a disease caused by plaques and tangles that develop within a person's brain, which lead to psychiatric symptoms initially but will eventually lead to that person's physiological death. It is a progressive neurological condition that moves through typical stages, although each person will express the symptoms a little differently and will progress through the stages at a different pace. The following will be a brief review of the stages and common presentations of each stage.

Early Stage of Dementia

In the early stage of Alzheimer's disease, the symptoms may be vague and not truly indicative of a problem. The mild changes in character and/or personality can be viewed as normal aging changes. This can be even more difficult to diagnose if a family member assists in compensating for the memory deficits of the individual. Initially, the person may present with mild short-term memory problems.

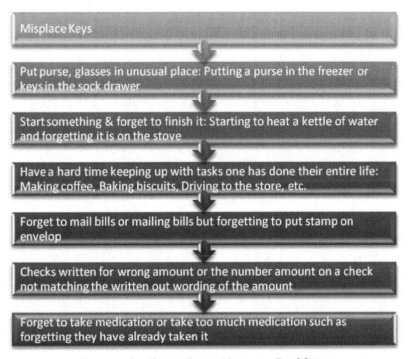

**Figure 13: Short-Term Memory Problems
in Early Alzheimer's Disease**

Tips for Communicating with a Person Suffering from Dementia

Caregivers can learn to communicate better with individuals suffering from dementia and improve their communication skills to help make caregiving less stressful. Good communication skills will also enhance their ability to handle the difficult behavior exhibited by individuals with a dementing illness.

Watch Body Language – The Person's and Yours: A caregiver's attitude and body language communicate feelings and thoughts stronger than words. Set a positive mood by speaking to a confused person in a pleasant and respectful manner. Use facial expressions, tone of voice and physical touch to help convey messages and show feelings of affection. If the person does not appear to understand what is being said, repeat the statement or question using different words. Talk slowly and in a monotone voice.

Get the person's attention: Limit distractions and noise – turn off all extraneous noise including the radio or TV, close the curtains or shut the door, or move to quieter surroundings. Before speaking, make sure the person is paying attention: use their name, identify yourself by name and relation, and use nonverbal cues and touch to help keep the person focused. If the person is seated, get down to the person's eye level and maintain eye contact.

Speak clearly: Use simple words and avoid the use of slang words or abstract terms. Talk in simple, direct sentences. Speak slowly, distinctly and in a reassuring tone. Refrain from speaking more loudly, because a person's voice may become higher-pitched when attempting to increase the volume, making it more difficult for the ill person to hear. Instead, when increasing the volume of your voice, use a lower tone so it is heard more easily i.e., make your voice deeper. If the person doesn't understand the first time, use the same wording to repeat what was said. If the person still doesn't understand, wait a few minutes and rephrase the question. Use the names of people and places instead of pronouns or abbreviations.

Ask simple, answerable questions: Ask one question at a time; limit questions which require yes or no answers – because often the answer will be 'no'. Refrain from asking open-ended questions or giving too many choices. For example, ask, *"Would you like to wear the red dress or the blue dress?"* Better still, show her the choices – visual prompts and cues also help clarify the question and can guide the response.

Listen with all of your senses: ears, eyes and heart: Be patient in waiting for a person to reply. If the person is struggling for an answer, it's okay to help and suggest words. Watch for nonverbal cues as well as body language, and respond appropriately. Always strive to listen for the meaning and feelings that underlie the words.

Break down activities into a series of steps: This makes many tasks much more manageable. Encourage the person to do what he/she can, gently reminding them of steps if the person tends to forget, and assist with steps the person is no longer able to accomplish on his/her own. Use visual cues, such as demonstrating how to put on a shirt and then allowing the person to do it themselves.

When the going gets tough, distract and redirect: When the person becomes upset, try changing the subject or the environment. For example, ask him for help or suggest deciding what's for dinner. *It is important to connect with the person on a feeling level, before attempting redirection techniques.* For example, 'I see you're feeling sad – I'm sorry you're upset. Let's go get something to eat.'

Respond with affection and reassurance: People suffering from dementia often feel confused, anxious and unsure of themselves. Further, they often get reality confused and may recall things that never really occurred. *Avoid trying to convince the person they are wrong.* Stay focused on the feelings they are demonstrating (which are real) and respond with verbal and physical expressions of comfort, support and reassurance. Sometimes holding hands, touching, hugging and praise will get the person to respond when all else fails.

Remember the good old days: Reminiscing about memories from the person's past is often a soothing and affirming activity. Many people with dementia may not remember what happened 45 minutes ago, but can clearly recall their lives 45 years earlier. Therefore, *avoid asking questions that rely on short-term memory,* such as asking the person what they had for lunch. Instead, try asking general questions about the person's distant past – when they were married or how many sisters or brothers the person had – this information is more likely to have been retained.

Maintain a sense of humor: *Use humor whenever possible; laugh with the person not at the person.* Most individuals with dementia tend to retain their social skills and are usually delighted to laugh along with you.

Handling Troubling Behavior

Some of the greatest challenges of caring for an individual with dementia are the personality and behavior changes that often occur. To meet these challenging situations, use creativity, flexibility, patience and compassion. It also helps to avoid taking things personally and maintain a sense of humor.

Understand that you cannot change the person: The person has a brain disorder that shapes who he/she has become. When caregivers attempt to control or change behaviors, most likely there will be failure or resistance. It's important to:

- *Try to accommodate the behavior, not control the behavior* – if the person insists on sleeping on the floor, place a mattress on the floor to make him/her more comfortable.
- *Remember that the caregiver* **can** *change their behavior or the physical environment but cannot change the person's.* Changing the caregiver's behavior will often result in a change in the confused person's behavior.

When there is a sudden change in behaviors or level of functioning (over a few hours to a few days) – there may be a cause other than the dementia: Behavioral problems may have an underlying medical problem: pain, constipation, an infection, or the person may be experiencing an adverse side effect from medications. In some cases, there may be some medication or treatment that can assist in managing the problem.

Some behaviors have a purpose: People with dementia typically have difficulty expressing themselves and cannot verbalize what they want or need. They might express their needs in another form – taking off their clothes or taking all of their shoes out of the closet on a daily basis, and caregivers wonder why. It may be that the person is fulfilling a need to be busy and productive. *Always consider what need the person might be trying to meet with their behavior – and, when possible, try to accommodate them.*

Some behaviors have a cause: It is important to understand that many behaviors have a cause or a trigger. It might be something a person did or said that triggered a behavior or it could be a change in the physical environment. *The root to changing behavior is disrupting the patterns that are causing the problematic behavior.* Try a different approach, or try a different way to react to a behavior.

Some things do not always work & What works today, May not tomorrow: Multiple factors will influence problematic behaviors and a dementia will progress, which means that solutions that are effective one day may need to be modified as time goes on – or the strategy may no longer work at all. The key to managing difficult behaviors is being creative and flexible in developing strategies to address a given issue.

Support – Learn from and share with others who have experience with these types of problems: Seek education, support groups, and talk to caregivers who have experience dealing with individuals suffering from dementia. It is difficult to obtain support from people who do not understand the ways a demented person can behave; people who have 'been there, seen that' can truly understand and

offer creative suggestions for developing strategies to help. Call the local Area Agency on Aging, the local chapter of the Alzheimer's Association, a Caregiver Resource Center, or search the internet for groups that can help. Expect that the person will have good days and bad days. Develop strategies for coping with the bad days.
(Family Caregiver Alliance, 2010)

Practical Tips in the Early Stage of Dementia

Individuals in the early stages of a dementia, including those suffering from Alzheimer's disease, may be able to live independently or live in their community with a relative or friend. Most are able to function adequately in the day-to-day activities of daily living. At this stage, it is wise to discuss the disease with the person, allow them to understand what is occurring and how the disease will progress so the person is able to make decisions on how he/she would like their care directed. Other helpful things would be to find ways to assist the person to live as independently as possible, for as long as possible.

Take Care of Business

While an individual is capable of making rational choices, encourage any person with a diagnosis of Alzheimer's disease, or any form of dementia, to make as many choices as possible regarding legal and medical decisions; this fosters independence and allows the person to have some say in their care. It is best if a person's wishes are detailed in writing so that there is no misunderstanding regarding a person's wishes. There are three very important documents to understand in determining the manner in which a person wishes his/her care to be directed: Living Will, Durable Power of Attorney, and Durable Financial Power of Attorney.

Living Will is a legal document that a person uses to make known his/her wishes regarding life prolonging medical measures. It has also been referred to as an advance directive, health care directive, or a healthcare provider's directive.

273

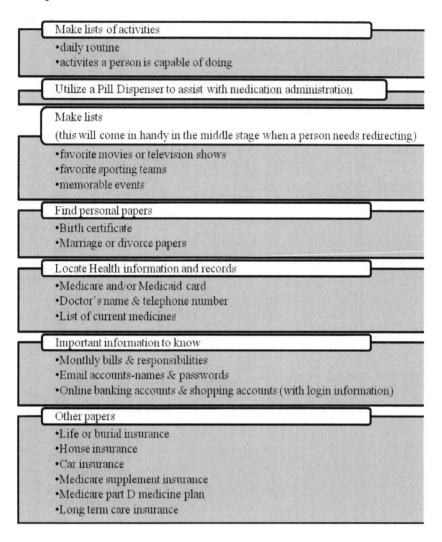

Make lists of activities
- daily routine
- activites a person is capable of doing

Utilize a Pill Dispenser to assist with medication administration

Make lists
(this will come in handy in the middle stage when a person needs redirecting)
- favorite movies or television shows
- favorite sporting teams
- memorable events

Find personal papers
- Birth certificate
- Marriage or divorce papers

Locate Health information and records
- Medicare and/or Medicaid card
- Doctor's name & telephone number
- List of current medicines

Important information to know
- Monthly bills & responsibilities
- Email accounts-names & passwords
- Online banking accounts & shopping accounts (with login information)

Other papers
- Life or burial insurance
- House insurance
- Car insurance
- Medicare supplement insurance
- Medicare part D medicine plan
- Long term care insurance

Figure 14: Practical Tips for the Early Stage of Dementia

It is important to have a living will as it informs a person's health care provider and their family about an individual's desires for medical treatment in the event he/she is not able to speak for him/herself (AllLaw.com, 2010). It is a lengthy document which presents multiple scenarios of health problems and asks the person to make decisions regarding their medical care. For example: 1) If you were diagnosed with Alzheimer's disease, you were in the late stages and were very confused, unable to communicate verbally, and were losing weight because you were unable to eat or drink a sufficient amount of food and fluids – would you want a feeding tube inserted to provide you with nutrition and hydration? 2) If you were diagnosed with a Stroke, were aware of your surroundings but unable to verbally communicate and unable to swallow without having problems – would you want a feeding tube inserted to provide you with nutrition and hydration? This document is completed, then a copy kept with the individual and/or relative, and a copy is filed with the medical provider directing the person's care.

Durable Power of Attorney is a document which assigns another individual to make medical decisions and authorizes that person to make financial decisions. This allows another person to make decisions regarding healthcare and to sign medical consent forms. This also allows the person access to an individual's bank accounts and finances, gives authority to sell property, and make decisions regarding the individual's living environment. A person with Alzheimer's disease authorizes this while he/she is legally capable of making decisions and the document is filed in a Court of Law in the county/state in which the person resides.

Durable Financial Power of Attorney is a document which authorizes another person to make only financial decisions. This allows another person access to bank accounts and finances and gives the person authority to sell property. The individual suffering from dementia authorizes this while he/she is legally capable of making decisions and the document filed in a Court of Law in the county/state in which the person resides.

Guardianship is another legal manner in which an individual who is unable to make decisions has another individual make decisions for him/her. If an individual is no longer competent to make decisions due to Alzheimer's disease or another disease process – and if there is no Advanced Directive or Durable Power of Attorney in place, and if there is no relative who is available to make decisions for the individual – the courts will assign a Guardian to make medical and financial decisions for the ill person. This is done to safeguard the individual and their personal property, including any income the person receives.

Caregivers

Those who care for any person who is cognitively impaired can have a difficult job that can be overwhelming at times. Each day can be challenging as a person's abilities decline or behaviors become problematic. Caregivers are at risk for depression and health problems caused by the stress of caring for another individual, especially if they have little support from family or friends. Some of the biggest struggles caregivers face involve dealing with difficult behaviors. Activities of daily living such as dressing, bathing, and eating often become difficult to manage for the person with a diagnosis of dementia, as well as the caregiver who assists in these activities. Developing a plan for getting through the day and a routine can assist caregivers cope. It is helpful to be creative and to develop strategies for dealing with difficult behaviors and stressful situations, though these strategies will not work every time (so it is good to search for alternative methods for managing). Through trial and error, caregivers will find what works and what does not. Each person with a diagnosis of dementia is unique and will respond differently to a given situation and may respond differently depending on the day and the person's mood, but it must be remembered that each person will change over the course of the disease (Caregiver Guide, 2010).

Life is full of burdens. Sometimes these burdens seem overwhelming...more than you feel you can handle. The good news is that you do not have to handle your burdens alone. You can rely on a power greater than yourself. Connect with others. Seek help and support.

Whether you call this means of strength God, Higher Power, or something else, recognize that you can seek help and guidance from this divine source. Connect with this spiritual power and share your burdens.

Recognize that you are not alone in anything you do.
Affirmations-AALTCN (2010)

Caregiver Survival Tips in the Early Stages of Dementia

Those who care for individuals suffering from dementia often take on a great deal of responsibility, which can be stressful emotionally, financially, and physically as the demands of caregiving takes its toll on a person. Acceptance of the diagnosis a person may have is the first step to survival. This will be followed by taking stock of the situation and educating oneself about the disease. Caregivers need to be educated on the disease: how a person will progress, common presentations, and ways to manage the behaviors to encourage independence and enhance quality of life for the person suffering from dementia. Caregivers must also be encouraged to seek support through support groups and medical providers. The following is a list of "things-to-do" for caregivers:

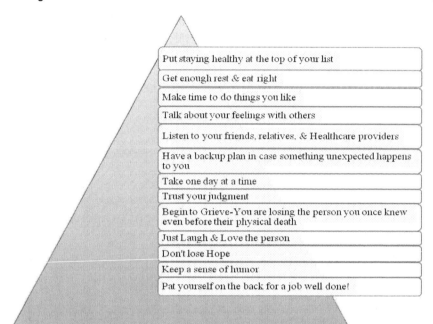

**Figure 15: Caregiver Survival Tips for the
Early Stages of Dementia**

Learn to say 'NO': There is no such thing as a perfect caregiver and caregivers must learn to say no in order to maintain their own sanity as well as that of the ill individual (at least as much as possible). Often, relatives and friends may not realize that having celebration dinners and holidays at an individual's residence can be stressful on the caregiver and upset the routine of a confused individual – which may be more problematic than anyone realizes.

One last thing on the "to-do" list: **GIVE YOURSELF PERMISSION TO MAKE MISTAKES**.

'If you've actively lived your life, been involved with others, and attempted to walk on unfamiliar paths, chances are you've made a fair share of mistakes.

Although mistakes can be hard – even painful – to go through, they offer a rich opportunity for growth. They give you insights that you may not have gotten otherwise. They also offer lessons about patience and forgiveness.

You certainly don't want to go out of your way to make mistakes, but when you do, accept them as important life lessons. Learn and grow from them.'

Affirmations-AALTCN (2010)

Making Memories

'A true friend Remembers for a Person
when their Memories fail them'

A person with any type of dementia, including Alzheimer's disease, will begin to lose their memories, initially the recent memories but, as time goes on and the disease progresses, most of these individuals will lose even their most remote memories. Make memories with the individual who has memory impairment as well as tap into the memories from the person's past while he/she can still share them. Spend time with the individual, have pictures taken of the individual, of family members with the individual as well as the individual with you. Find old pictures and ask the individual to tell you names, dates, and circumstances surrounding the picture AND write this information on the back of the photograph. Pictures of the person as a child are some of the most enjoyable memories for most older individuals. Also locate personal memorabilia such as old love letters, drawings by grandchildren, old baby booties, dried flowers, or old pieces of jewelry. Ask the person to share a story about the item and write these stories down on a note card. Take all of these items and create a memory box – it does not have to be expensive – an old shoe box or cigar box will do, just keep the memory box handy for use when an individual becomes agitated or fixated on doing something inappropriate or going somewhere that is not in the person's best interest. When these circumstances occur, pull out the photos or Memory box, start talking about the story surrounding the memory and hopefully you will tap into the person's memory and this will offer some distraction, draw his/her attention away from what has caused him/her to be agitated, allow an individual to reminisce and calm a confused, agitated individual.

Communication Tips

The following tips may help anyone who wishes to communicate with an individual with confusion or dementia:

- Decrease excessive noise in the environment by turning off TV or Radio before talking
- Keep conversations or requests short & simple, but not childlike
- Be patient
- Give lots of time for a person to answer a question
- If a person losses train of thought, either repeat the same question again or ask the question a little differently
- Give lots of time for a person to finish what they are saying, even if they ramble
- Don't butt in
- Don't fill in the missing words unless a person says it's okay
- Pay close attention to body language – both theirs and yours
- If you guess at what is being said, ask if your guess is right
- If a person can't say what they mean, ask them to point to it
- REMEMBER, often you cannot change a person with dementia; it is your job to change the way YOU talk to this person!

Early Dementia: Enhancing Eating

The following are tips to avoid eating problems or improve the life of an individual with dementia or who is in the early stages of Alzheimer's disease:

- Offer to cook meals for the person or have meals delivered
- Assist with shopping trips to the grocery store – be cognizant of the type of foods you buy:
  - Easy to make foods
  - Sandwich materials
  - Water
- Check for foods gone bad as a person with Alzheimer's disease loses their sense of smell
- Call or drop by to see if the person has eaten (or remind them to eat)
- Leave a note by the phone reminding a person to eat
- Ask a neighbor to drop by around lunch time to remind the ill person to eat
- Meals on Wheels or church delivery group can also assist

Problems in the Middle Stage of Dementia

In the middle stage of a dementia, such as Alzheimer's disease, there can be more behavioral problems since a person is 'forgetting they forget' and begins to believe some of the things their minds are telling them inaccurately. This stage can last 2 to 10 years. They may begin to have difficulty walking, trouble sitting down & getting up from a seated position, trouble going to the bathroom (such as urinating or having a bowel movement), trouble finding their way around the house (or getting lost in familiar places), trouble getting dressed, or having difficulty dealing with noise, lights, & crowds (overstimulating environments).

Commonly, in the middle stages, an individual may no longer read (some have said they get lost in reading or forget what the 1st part of paragraph was discussing), cannot keep up with movies or television shows due to an inability to remember characters or plots of stories, become unable to recognize words or unable to recognize what words mean, may have trouble making sense of telephone messages since they do not realize the person is not in the same room, develop trouble using cues such as notes & reminders,

281

may have trouble eating (either forget they are eating or forget the steps of eating – needing cues to start eating, chew, swallow, or possibly drink), may have trouble finding words or putting thoughts together, and often have trouble living independently.

The following are common problematic behaviors exhibited in the middle stage of Alzheimer's disease:

- Makes up stories as memory fails but the person believes the story to be true
- Confuses who people are or their relationship; May think family members are strangers
- Sleeps more during daytime; may wake up through the night (Days & Nights mixed up)
- Tell the same story over & over
- Ask the same questions over & over
- Talks but the words don't make sense
- Argues with the caregiver about tasks such as bathing or changing soiled clothes
- Fidgets with things; pill-rolling with hands; rocking with body
- Walks constantly; Wanders
- Tries to leave the house to go 'home'
- Becomes extremely anxious and nervous in the afternoon & evening hours (Sundowning)
- Trouble differentiating 'what is real' from 'what is not real'
- Begins to see & hear things that are not there
- Possibly develops delusions i.e., convinces self husband is cheating; convinced that someone is stealing her purse
- May become combative during tasks of daily living such as hits, bites, or pushes you away

Home Safety

There are normal aging changes in individuals that can cause safety problems. There is a yellowing of the lens of the eyes which can make certain colors (such as blues, greens, and purples) more difficult to see while other colors (such as reds, oranges, and yellows) are seen more clearly. Objects in close proximity, that are similar in color, can blend and become lost – use contrasting colors so objects are seen more clearly – such as contrasting colored plates and table. Busy patterns in rugs, wallpaper, or on furniture can make an individual off balance or confused – solid colors or simple patterns are encouraged. Loose rugs can be a fall hazard due to arthritic changes in individuals, so double sided tape on the bottom of rugs can prevent slips or falls.

Ways to make the world of an Individual with Dementia safer include:
- Make their world simple
- Use plain colored placemats, bath towels & sheets
- Block off stairs to prevent falls (i.e., use a toddler gate)
- Have all locks keyed to same key (do not leave key in the lock); turn bolt locks can allow an individual to open the lock and wander outside
- On doors to the outside – place latches up too high or too low for an individual to reach
- Have person wear an ID bracelet provided by the Alzheimer's Association's Safe Return Program
- Lock cabinets and drawers containing knives, sharp objects, soaps, cleaners, poison and medicines
- During sunny times of day, glare can cause problems – pull down blinds or close curtains in the evening
- Make sure string pulls on blinds are wrapped around a hook as high on the wall as an individual can reach to prevent the arms & legs of the person from becoming tangled in these strings
- Consider changing glass windows in the bathroom/bedrooms to thick plastic

Communication Tips in the Middle Stages of Dementia:
- Sometimes when an individual is disoriented and reorientation may not be appropriate due to impairment of short term memory:
  - Do not try to reorient – this can cause agitation & arguments

283

- Better: Use distraction (change the subject) & redirection (divert his/her attention)

■ Individuals suffering from dementia may need cues to perform tasks
  - Do not give a series of instructions ('Let's get dressed')
  - Better: Give one cue or instruction at a time ('Put your shirt on,' then wait for the individual to put on the shirt)

■ Speak directly to the person and look directly at him/her to ensure you are heard

■ Speak slowly and in a calm tone of voice

■ Look at the person's body language – what is it saying
  - BOTH YOURS AND THEIRS

■ Limit Choices
  - Do not give open ended choices ('What do you want to wear today?')
  - Better: Offer 2 or 3 choices to prevent confusion to enlist cooperation ('Do you want to wear the red shirt or the blue one?')

■ Be patient & calm

■ Touch is very important

■ Don't talk to the person like he/she is a child or use baby talk

■ Stop what you are doing – really listen to what the person is saying

■ Think about the feelings behind the words

■ If person looks angry or upset – ask why

■ Treat the person with dignity & respect

■ Say exactly what you want the person to do

■ Use ordinary words
  - Bad – 'hop in bed'
  - Better – 'please get in the bed'

■ Don't ask yes/no questions: Turn your questions into answers for person
  - Bad – 'do you need to go to the bathroom?'

- Better – 'the bathroom is right over there, I can walk with you.'

■ **Do's & Don'ts**
  - Do take a deep breath
  - Do be patient
  - Do be creative
  - Do allow the person to make as many decisions as possible
  - Do listen to what the person is saying
  - Do show respect for the person
  - Don't ignore the person
  - Don't argue
  - Don't try to rationalize with an irrational person
  - Don't correct or fuss at a person for getting something wrong
  - Don't say 'I just told you that'
  - Don't ask the person to 'remember' things (they probably do not remember)
  - Don't say 'You can't do that by yourself'; Better: 'Do as much as you can and I will help you'
  - Don't be too demanding
  - Don't try to make the person see things from your point of view – this ability is gone

Other Factors to Consider

Crowds can be upsetting & confusing and increase agitation. Try to limit the number of guests in the house at one time or have guests talk with the individual away from the crowd and noise. If the person gets upset, move to a quiet area with the person until he/she calms down.

Routine is very important for individuals with Alzheimer's disease or any type of dementia. Establish a daily routine in order to allow the confused person to feel some degree of accomplishment. Upsetting their daily routine can result in problematic behaviors. Aim for consistency in:

- Environment
- Caregivers
- Meal time
- Bathing/showering schedule
- Elimination: Routine toileting for urination as well as bowel movements
- Nap schedule

Allow repetition in the person's routine:

- The person may wish to wear the same style of clothes or the same outfit every day
- The person may wish to eat the same foods frequently
- The person may wish to watch their favorite TV shows or movies repeatedly
- Exercise: same activities every day
- May talk about their favorite things – over and over

Activities That can be Difficult for Confused Individuals

Dressing:

- Lay clothes out in the order the person puts them on – do not stack the clothes (lay them out side by side in the order the person will dress)
- Offer one piece of clothing at a time for the person to put on
- Give cues – 'here is your shirt'
  - Possibly demonstrate how to put on the shirt
- Set aside time for the person to dress (this allows the person to be more independent and feel a sense of accomplishment)
- Use Praise: Tell the person they are doing a good job
- If the person wants to wear the same clothes over & over – let them; try buying more clothes that look alike

Toileting

- Mark the path to bathroom clearly
- Establish a way to make the location of the bathroom noticeable
  - May use a sign: 'BATHROOM'

- Put picture of toilet on door
- Watch for cues like fidgeting with clothes or pacing
- Write down the time of day the person has 'accidents' so you can schedule toileting to prevent incontinent episodes
- Timed toileting: a routine schedule of taking the person to the bathroom and encouraging the person to try to urinate: walk to bathroom every 2 to 3 hours
  - Do not wait for person to ask
- Limit fluids 2 to 3 hours before bedtime and have person toilet immediately before going to bed

Mouth Care
- Daily mouth care
- Step-by-step instructions
  - It's time to brush your teeth
  - Come with me
  - We're going to the bathroom to brush your teeth
  - I will help you
  - Here is the toothpaste
  - Take off the top
  - Squeeze the toothpaste on the brush
  - You're doing a great job!

Bathing
- Gather every item necessary for bathing ahead of time
  - Towel, bath mat, soap, shampoo, comb, lotion, powder
- Make sure the room is warm enough
- Make sure the water temperature is adequate and test the water temperature
- Use hand-held shower sprayer
  - Overhead spraying from a showerhead can be a source of anxiety for confused individuals
- Consider using a shower bench for the person to sit on
- Don't bath too often due to skin dryness of older individuals

- Bathing 2 to 3 times a week is plenty unless the person is having frequent toileting accidents
- Tell the person what is happening one step at a time
- Invite the person to help
- Give the person a washcloth even if they cannot help wash
- Help the person cover his/her face with a towel when you wash his/her hair – keeps water from getting in a person's eyes
- Maintain privacy – keep the person covered
  - Lay towel across lap or chest
  - Use washcloth to clean under towel
- If the person gets upset about getting wet, start at feet and slowly move up
- Offer distraction – try talking, singing, or asking person to hold the soap

Sleeping

- Hallucinations or delusions
  - Keep a small light on in the room – especially if a person is afraid of the dark
  - Shadows can be seen as hallucinations
  - Help prevent falls with night lights and by removing unnecessary clutter in the path to the bathroom to assist in preventing falls due to toileting at nighttime
  - Diminish clutter to decrease confusing a disoriented person
- Fear
  - Due to the person seeing or hearing things that are not really there
  - Sit with the person to calm and assure them
  - Do not argue with the person that the hallucination is not real
- Temperature
  - Check if the room is too warm or cool
- Offer distractions
  - Try 'white noise'
    - » Hum of a fan or soft music

» Avoid music with a lot of words or a radio station that has people talking frequently
- Hunger may cause a person to get up through the night seeking something to eat
  - Offer a snack at least an hour before bedtime
- Too many daytime naps may cause a person to be up at nighttime
  - Limit daytime napping if the person is frequently wandering at night (may be getting too much sleep)
  - Also remember, if the person is overly tired – he/she may also have trouble staying asleep at night

Common Triggers for Agitation in Confused Individuals
- Asking a person to do more than he/she is capable
- Having too much noise or activity
- Changing where a person lives
- Having too many people around
- Planning bath time
- Asking a person to change clothes

Ways to manage an upset confused individual
- Identify the behavior or action that is problematic
- Ask the person: What has upset you? Are you hurt? Can I help? I am sorry (even if you didn't do anything)
- Try to identify what triggered the behavior
  - Where did the behavior happen?
  - What happened right before the behavior started?
  - Check for pain, hunger, thirst, constipation, full bladder, tiredness/fatigue
  - Check for clothes that are too tight or too loose
- Identify ways to manage problematic behaviors and attempt this same technique the next time the behavior presents

Helpful Hints
- Stay calm
- Take the upset person to another, quiet place

- Redirection: Enlist the person to do something by asking in simple, direct language, change the subject
- Listen to what the person is saying
- Try to understand what is going on – from the person's point of view
- Use a quiet tone of voice
- Do not get upset about the behavior – this will escalate the problem
- Check for pain, hunger, thirst, constipation, full bladder, tiredness/fatigue
- Check for clothes that are too tight or too loose
- Try using art, music, or touch to help relax the person
- Use some form of distraction: Get out a memory book or treasure box that you have put together
  - Use pictures or items to talk about good memories
- Take a walk, play ball, or go for a car ride
- **Things to do & Things not to do**
  - Do say comfort words
    - » May I help you?
    - » You're safe here
    - » Everything is under control
    - » I am sorry – apologize
    - » I'm sorry that you are upset
    - » I know it's hard
    - » I will stay until you feel better
  - **Do Not**
    - » Raise voice
    - » Argue or try to reason with the person who is disoriented
    - » Try to grab or corner the person
    - » Show you are afraid
    - » Let the person hurt your feelings

Eating Problems

- Verify there is no problem with teeth or gums
  - Take the person to a dentist to rule out: Sore gums, caries, broken teeth, or poor fitting dentures

- Establish a routine: Serve meals at the same time every day
- Serve foods with different colors & textures
- Make the dining table a calm place to eat
- Use plain colored dishes that are different from the color of the food
  - Avoid dishes with patterns – may be too confusing
- Use a shallow bowl with a lip to prevent food from being pushed off the plate
- Put only the fork or spoon that is needed to eat next to the plate
- Take things like sauces, ketchup bottles, or salt & pepper off table
  - Too confusing
- Remind the person to eat & drink
- Consider offering 4 to 5 small meals plus snacks instead of 3 meals a day

If a Confused Person refuses to eat
- Possible causes
  - Too many choices
  - Trouble initiating eating
  - Trouble remembering how to eat
- Helpful hints
  - Offer one food at a time
  - Demonstrate to the person how to eat
  - Finger foods
    » Offer high protein snacks
    » Provide high protein foods that can be eaten on the go
    » Put anything between 2 slices of bread
  - Offer more choices of fresh fruits & vegetables
  - Soft foods
    » Consider chopping meats or puree foods
  - Play soft music unless this seems to cause more distraction
  - Don't rush the person during eating periods
  - Keep a list of foods the person will eat

291

- Try sweet, salty, sour or spicy foods/seasonings
- Check to see if a person has swallowed the last bite before proceeding with eating
- Try ice cream, thick soups or milkshakes with an egg, protein mix, or Carnation® Breakfast added to them

Behavior	Common Triggers	Helpful hints	Things NOT to do
Suspicion	• Mistaking what a person sees or hears • Losing or misplacing things • Forgetting where a person is	• Let a person know he/she is safe & that you care • Listen to a person's point of view • Listen to the feelings behind the words • Give a person a simple answer • Offer help to find what is missing or lost • If a person keeps losing the same item over & over » Have several of the same items i.e. wallets, purses, toothbrushes, glasses, favorite shirt • Provide a person with what is lost then distract person • If a person keeps asking when someone will return or when they can leave: Ask the	• Raise your voice • Get angry or upset • Argue or try to reason with disoriented person

Behavior	Common Triggers	• Helpful Hints	Things NOT to do
Suspicion (continued)		person when he/she believes the person will be back or when the person believes he/she can leave	
Aggression	• Your emotions • Anxiety • Feelings of threat • Feeling out of control • Too much noise • Too many people	• Stay calm • Be safe • Respect a person's personal space • Stay at an arm's length – it hurts less if you are hit from a distance as opposed to up close • If a person does not wish to do something, give a person some time & try again later	• Shout back • Demand an explanation • Put your hands on your hips, frown, or point your finger at person – watch body language • Get too close, so a person feels crowded • Make a person feel threatened
Hallucina-tions	• Patterns on walls, rugs, or furniture • Shadows due to poor lighting or night-time • Reflections in mirrors or windows	• Reassure the person • Respond calmly • Touch person or tap a person gently on shoulder to turn a person's focus back on you • Look for feelings that caused the person to see or hear things that aren't there • Say 'it sounds as if you're worried' or 'I know this frightens you'	• Argue • Ignore a person's feelings

Behavior	Common Triggers	Helpful hints	Things NOT to do
Hallucina-tions (continued)		• Suggest taking a walk or sitting in another room • See that the room is well lighted • Try to redirect or focus on music or another activity • Check for noises from TV or an air conditioner • Look for lighting that casts shadows • Cover mirrors or close window blinds	
Repetitive Behaviors	• Short-term memory loss • Anxiety • Boredom • Depression	• Stay calm & be patient • Reassure the person in a calm voice & gentle touch • Look for a reason behind behavior & remove it if possible • Turn the action or behavior into an activity • If rubbing hand across table, give person a cloth to help with dusting • Give a person the answer they are looking for, even if you have to repeat it several times	• Raise your voice • Tell person you have already answered the question • Ignore the person • Demand that the person stop

Behavior	Common Triggers	Helpful hints	Things NOT to do
Repetitive Behaviors (continued)		• Ask the person to answer the question i.e., repeat the question back to the person • Use reminder props such as notes	• Tell the person they are making you crazy
Wandering	• Stress • Confusion to time • Restlessness • Agitation • Anxiety Inability to recognize familiar people, places, or objects • Possibly: Medication side effects	• Keep recent photographs or videotape of the person to show police if the person becomes lost • Keep all doors secured • Consider a keyed deadbolt • Use safety latches up high or very low on doors leading to the outside (so the person cannot reach it) • Have the person wear an identification bracelet • Make sure the person gets enough exercise & sleep • Let the person do chores: Fold cloths, or help with setting the table, etc.	• Raise your voice • Restrain the person • Lock the person in a room • Leave the person alone • Give a person a sedative to stop the wandering behavior, unless there is risk of injury to the person or another

Behavior	Common Triggers	Helpful hints	Things NOT to do
Wandering (continued)		• Cover door knobs with cloth or paint them the same color as the wall – so the person will not notice the knob • Keep a current picture of the person • Remember what color clothes the person is wearing on a daily basis in case you must try to seek assistance from others to help find the person who has wandered away	

Helpful Hints for Day-to-Day Tasks

Eating: Keep mealtime calm and comfortable; offer one food at a time; try different or new foods; make foods visible – not similar in color to the plate; be aware of foods on which a person can choke; use straws or cups with lids or handles; try finger foods – preferably high in protein; offer healthy snacking; allow enough time for meals and allow the person to be as independent as possible – allow him/her to feed self as long as possible; and monitor weight.

Dressing: Encourage independence; organize clothes in the order the person will put them on; demonstrate how to put on the clothes if necessary but allow the person to do it him/herself; choose comfortable, simple clothes; limit choices – 2 to 3 choices to prevent the person from being overwhelmed by choices; and keep a routine – getting dressed at the same time of day so the person can be familiar with the routine.

Bathing: Try showers and baths to see what method works best for that particular person; be prepared with all supplies necessary for bathing; have the person assist in the bath as much as possible; be aware of water temperature; daily baths are not necessary for older individuals – bathing 2 to 3 times a week may be adequate as long as the person appears (and smells) clean and there are no skin issues; be safe – use shower benches and bath mats to prevent falls; be gentle – an older person's skin is often dryer and can tear easily; and use lotion to prevent overly drying skin.

Toileting: Remind the person to use the toilet – consider times for toileting; every 2 to 3 hours for individuals who may be incontinent (be cautious in asking the person if he/she needs to toilet – the answer to a yes/no question is often NO even if the person really does need to urinate); monitor bowel movement to prevent constipation (many times, bowel movements will occur after meals – especially breakfast – and after a stimulating beverage such as coffee, tea, or prune juice); provide a clear path to the bathroom (no rugs, furniture, or objects which block the path); consider rubber mats near the toilet if the person has incontinence as well as rubber sheets (under linen sheets) to protect the mattress, and incontinence pads; learn the person's routine (the most common times for an episode of urinary incontinence); avoid caffeinated drinks (cola, coffee, tea, and chocolate); and limit fluids 2 hours prior to bedtime (and have the person void immediately before going to bed).

Communicating: Be comforting and reassuring; be patient; show the person you are interested; try not to criticize or correct; offer a guess if you do not understand – ask questions and repeat what they are saying to let them know you are paying attention; look at the feelings behind the words; ask for nonverbal communication (pointing or gestures); use short, simple sentences; give one instruction at a time; use the person's name; speak slowly and clearly; repeat information and questions if the person does not seem to understand; identify objects by name or – if the person does not seem to understand – use a different name to refer to the object; do not use abstract terms; do not use negative terms such as 'Don't do that' – instead use positive terms such as 'why don't we do this'; give the person a choice in limited forms, do not ask open ended questions – 'What would you like to wear today?' – Instead ask 'Would you like to wear the red outfit or the blue outfit?'; if the person is not responding – try again later; watch your tone of voice and body language; and use body language and gestures to convey what you are asking (Alzheimer's Activities Guide, 2005).

Therapeutic Activities for Individuals with Dementia

Individuals with dementia benefit greatly from structured, individualized activities that involve and interest the person. These activities may reduce many of the problematic behaviors including agitation, anger, frustration, depression, wandering or rummaging. Therapeutic activities should focus on the person's previous interests, cue the person to old and recent memories and take advantage of the person's remaining skills while minimizing the impact of skills that may be compromised (Fisher, 2010). The basis of individualized care can be based on a technique called the Montessori method.

Montessori Method

Caregivers can utilize the Montessori techniques in their interactions with individuals with dementia. In structuring their routine and developing activities, there are five underlying guidelines for relating to people with dementia:

* An activity or experience should support a sense of self-worth by allowing the person to feel like they are contributing to society, community, or the household
* Individuals should have an opportunity to express their thoughts and feelings
* Individuals must have a sense of accomplishment and success
* Individuals should experience a sense of inclusion and belonging, being part of a group or family
* Individuals must have a sense of routine and order; it is vital that they feel comfortable and secure within established boundaries which create a safe environment

(Keane, 2003)

Try to plan all activities using familiar, real-life materials. Begin with simple, one-step activities (use inexpensive things like rice, chickpeas, or kidney beans, which are easy to scoop, for activities) and, as the person is able to increase the difficulty, move to other activities that are more complex. As a person's skills develop, facilitators will begin to pursue another major Montessori principle, which is to move the activity from a concrete experience to something in the abstract. A small group might be involved in flower arranging which is a simple skill activity; in the course of the activity, the facilitator and the individual with a diagnosis of dementia move to a discussion about flowers, which is a type of reminiscence activity. The facilitator might say, 'Susie, why do you keep choosing those particular flowers to put in the vase? What do the flowers remind you of?' Then Susie might respond with a memory from her past, a beautiful story of how her mother loved flowers (Keane, 2003).

Many individuals with dementia find it difficult to verbalize what they wish to communicate or have difficulties relaying their feelings; it is important to provide an alternative form of communication through demonstration. A structured atmosphere that is more physical – expression-dominated rather than speech-dominated – creates an environment conducive to learning for these individuals. Another important principle is to have actions move in a defined direction, an order in which the activity will occur-from left to right, top to bottom – and to consistently use that approach with the group to reinforce natural patterns. For example, when assisting a person in dressing, lay clothes out in the order they should be put on, from left to right. Or when having a flower arranging activity, place the vase, then flowers, and then ribbons or any other items used for this activity in the order in which they will be used.

All activities should be broken down into individualized steps – from a larger context to a smaller context, making it easier for the person to comprehend. For example, a treasure hunt – a simple container is filled with navy beans through which a person must dig to retrieve hidden items. As self-esteem and confidence grow through success, this simple 'hunt and find' activity can be adapted to a small group of two persons suffering from dementia: Set out a checkerboard and hide the checkers in the bean-filled container. One person digs through the beans, grabs a checker, and gives it to the other person who places it on the checkerboard. These types of activities, which are broken down into individual steps performed by a small team, helps individuals with dementias to develop and/or maintain motor skills helpful in other aspects of their lives, such as eating or dressing (Keane, 2003).

Guidelines for Choosing Therapeutic Activities

There are a variety of activities appropriate for people at every stage of their dementia. Keep in mind that doing an activity is more important than the end result – even if the person was a perfectionist or very goal directed before the onset of their disease. Performing an activity has its own rewards and benefits.

Guidelines for Therapeutic Activities

* Individualized activities which draw upon past interests and skills
* Choose activities that recall the person's former occupation
* Stimulate the 5 senses: sight, hearing, taste, touch, smell
* Use existing physical skills
* Help the person by initiating the activity (and helping along if necessary)
* Ensure the activity is voluntary
* Select intergenerational activities
* Choose activities that appeal to both the facilitator and the person with dementia
* Keep activities short

What kinds of therapeutic activities are best?

Activities should support a person's sense of self and bring out their skills, memories and habits as well as reinforce the person's sense of being in a group, which can provide friendship, mutual support and connectedness with their surroundings. There are a number of activities that may be beneficial depending on the person and their level of functioning, and different activities may affect certain symptoms but not others. For example, Music therapy may improve eating in some people but not others. It is preferable to plan activities the person would have enjoyed when they were younger, to play on the person's remote memory. For example, any former hobby or interest from gardening, cooking, painting and drawing, to singing, playing musical instruments or listening to music, etc. Developing a structured routine is essential: Activities that are done regularly, perhaps even at the same time every day if possible, may help establish routine and increase the person's sense of stability (Fisher, 2003).

Several programs that combine various therapeutic activities have also shown favorable results in people suffering from dementia. These include a multifaceted program of music, exercise, crafts and

301

relaxation, and structured sessions combining meditation, relaxation, sensory awareness and guided imagery, and so-called mind-over-body techniques designed to calm and soothe (Keane, 2003).

Many of the activities described below can be found in the 'Alzheimer's Activity Guide: In it Together'

Outings

Going places with people who are suffering from dementia is important and keeps them connected with the world around them as well as helps them feel like they are still a part of a community. Unfamiliar places can be confusing and upsetting to individuals with dementia. It is important to structure any outing so the person is not overwhelmed and the outing is conducive to their enjoyment.

Sporting events: If professional games are too expensive, consider amateur games such as minor league baseball, high school or college games. There may be less pressure in buying the ticket, finding parking, or dealing with crowds. And if the person is not having a good day, it will be less frustrating to change plans. If a live event is too stressful for a person, consider watching the sporting event on television or listening to a radio broadcast.

Zoo: Seeing exotic animals can be enjoyable; ask the person if he/she would like to see any particular animal. Limit the initial excursions to one or two less crowded sections of the zoo and consider the petting zoo as long as it is not too crowded. Touching animals and having real interaction can make the person feel connected with society and help with reminiscing about pleasant memories. Be aware of the animal's reaction to the person so not to frighten the person. If a trip to the zoo is too stressful, bring an animal to visit the person – a cat or dog which is friendly and calm. If the person is not apprehensive and reacts favorably, allow the person to pet the animal. Also walking a pet is good exercise and can be more pleasant than walking alone for individuals with dementia. Consider a stuffed animal or doll for contact with what the person may believe is real.

Art Museum: Visits to art museums can be visually stimulating as well as relaxing. Many museums have interactive exhibits so the person can touch some of the art. Walk through the exhibits and ask the person about their thoughts and feelings about the artwork. Discuss colors and any subjects triggered by the visit. Consider bringing a wheelchair if the person gets too tired from walking. If a visit to an art museum is too stressful, consider excursions to a library to look at art books or bring art books to the person. Set up pictures in a room of the house and stage an exhibit.

Fruit picking: When choosing the location, pick one that is not too physically demanding for the person. Avoid fruit trees which require a ladder to get to the fruit or fruits that have sharp thorns such as blackberries or raspberries. Consider strawberry or blueberry farms or an orchard with smaller trees. Consider going to a fruit stand and allowing the person to help pick out the fruits and vegetables to bring home and then wash them together. Also elicit the person's ideas for making fruit pies or fruit salad. Consider a small garden in the backyard or potted plants on tables that are easy to reach.

Bowling: Stimulates hand-eye coordination and can be fun as well as foster team spirit. Bowling may help balance problems also. Help lift the ball and allow the person to assist with guiding it down the alley. Make sure the game is not competitive or ask the bowling alley to put up the bumpers for the gutter and use the lightest ball. If bowling is too stressful, the person may wish to go to the bowling alley and watch, and then have discussions about the game.

Kite flying: An inexpensive kite or one which you make can be visually stimulating and allow the person to enjoy the outdoors.

Be mindful of safety – watch the weather, be careful about power-lines, never use a kite with metallic parts, and be aware of fall or tripping hazards. Consider getting the kite in the air and then allowing the person to hold the string. If flying the kite is too stressful, bring a comfortable chair for the person to sit in and watch the kite flying.

Boat watching: Going to a local area to watch boats can be a very relaxing activity. Be mindful of safety around water.

Library: Looking at, reading, or simply touching books can be stimulating. Reading a book together or listening to a recorded narrative of a book, one on CD or audio cassette, is also enjoyable. Some libraries offer special events for elders. If the person has difficulty reading and comprehending, books with large pictures may be an alternative. Find a quiet comfortable area to avoid distractions. Ask the person questions about the story or pictures while reading.

Visiting family/friends: A short visit to see family members or friends is a pleasurable activity which allows the person to interact with others as well as get out of the house. Being in familiar places may help trigger memories and stimulate conversations. If going out is too stressful, riding in the car around the block or having family and friends come visit the person may be enjoyable. Make sure visitors are aware of the person's limitations and have visitors come in 1 to 3 people at one time, direct conversations to include the person, and do not carry on multiple conversations in the same room as the person.

Crafts & Hobbies

Helping create something can be extremely satisfying. This type of activity can foster hand-eye coordination and help maintain a person's motor skills. It can also tap into a person's creativity.

<u>Visiting a Craft Show</u>: Craft shows are great for interacting with others, can stimulate all of the senses, and are a good way for persons with dementia to explore. Once at the show, allow the person to wander from table to table (with supervision) and discuss the things a person is seeing. If going to a show would be too stressful or difficult, bring home craft magazines, how-to books, or things a person would see at a craft's show and have one at home.

<u>Pressing flowers & leaves</u>: This is a creative activity which combines physical activity, contact with nature, and using visual skills. Gather leaves and/or flowers from a nature walk but avoid moldy or rotten ones – making sure the leaves are dry, press them between two sheets of newspaper and place heavy books on top, and allow them to flatten for 24 hours (flowers usually require 3 days). If you wish, next take wax paper, place the flower or leaf between the sheets and press with a warm iron for 10 seconds, but care should be taken so the person does not hurt themself or burn anything. Flowers may need to be refrigerated prior to use.

<u>Making a mobile</u>: Gather several lightweight objects of similar shape and size (such as shells, buttons, and/or beads), a lightweight string, and a plastic hanger. Tie the string around each object, leaving 6 inches of string on top, and allow the person to tie the object to the hanger. The person can continue to add objects until he/she decides the mobile is complete. If the activity is too stressful, make a mobile and allow the person to choose the order and placement of the objects. Use caution with small objects which can be placed in a person's mouth and lead to choking.

<u>Stringing beads for bracelets or necklaces</u>: Use sturdy string and large colorful beads that easy to handle, but be careful the person does not put the beads in their mouth. Use a tape measure to measure the wrist or neck and make the string 6 inches longer than you measure. Cut string, tie a one bead on the end – 3 inches from

305

the end of the string, and then allow the person to add beads. You may need to demonstrate how to perform the task. If the activity is too stressful, allow the person to choose the colors and the order in which the beads are placed on the string. Some individuals can work with others who have dementia which creates a partnership as well as fosters interaction with others (it will be dependent on the level of functioning for both individuals).

<u>Making a birdfeeder</u>: All you need to make a birdfeeder are sturdy string, a pinecone, peanut butter, and birdseed. Tie a string at the top of the pinecone, apply peanut butter to the pinecone, and allow the person to roll the peanut butter pinecone in the birdseed. Place the pinecone where the person can watch the birds come feed if possible. If this activity is too stressful for the person, talk through the steps and ask the person where the birdfeeder should be placed, preferably where the person can watch the birds come to feed. Talk about what kind of birds will come.

<u>Creating a collage</u>: Gather safety scissors, photographs, sturdy board or corkboard, and a glue stick. Try to include pictures of family members, friends, or animals. As you put the collage together, discuss who the people in the pictures are – if the person is having difficulties recalling who they are, provide hints to trigger remote memories. If this activity is too stressful, allow the person to direct which pictures are used, where to place them, and talk about who they are.

<u>Arranging flowers</u>: Gather all necessary are flowers and a vase – scissors are optional – you may cut the ends of the stems prior to having the person help. Allow the person to pick which flowers to use and the placement. If this is too stressful, allow the person to pick which flowers to place in the vase or talk about the flowers as you arrange them in a vase. Put the flower arrangement where the person can see it after completion of the activity.

Making a picture frame: A homemade picture frame is creative and a constructive activity. They can be used by the person or given as a gift. To make one – obtain an inexpensive frame, use glue and attach buttons, shells, paperclips, peas, or any small objects to the front of the frame (making sure the person does not place the objects in their mouth). Allow the frame to dry and then insert a photo of something or someone of significance for the person after completion of the activity. Colorful pictures from a magazine can also be used. If this is too stressful for the person, allow the person to direct you on what is put on the frame and where they are placed; the person can decide when the project is complete.

Playing with modeling clay or Play-Doh©: Get non-toxic modeling clay, which comes in a variety of colors, to allow the person to use to create something. Allow the person to decide what to make but if they do not have any ideas, suggestions can include paperweights, cups, coin bowls, etc. Play-Doh is softer than modeling clay and may be easier to work with. If this is too stressful, allow the person to direct what is made and place the object they designed where they can see it. Use caution to assure the person does not eat the clay.

Making Holiday cards: Encourage the person to design a card, including the design, and the words for the card. Offer suggestions and you may need to talk them through the activity. While making the card, talk about past holidays and the people to whom the card will be sent. If the person has difficulty writing, ask them what to include or allow them to choose from a few pre-thought out ideas.

Music

Music can be enjoyable, stimulate memory, and enhance verbal and visual skills. It can contribute to resynchronization (the stimulation of the timing processes within the brain) which can assist in improving the timing of motor actions including walking or swinging arms.

307

Singing songs: Give a copy of the lyrics to the person and encourage him/her to sing along with the singing or music. It may be helpful to offer the person one sheet of music at a time. If this is too stressful or the person cannot read any longer, just play the music and sing for them.

Going to concerts: Look for concerts or music events which are of interest for the person; many are free as well as many school choirs and church groups will offer free concerts for elders. If the person is unable to attend a concert, find a CD or tape of music the person would enjoy.

Playing a musical instrument: If a person played a musical instrument, ask if he/she would like to play again. Ask the person to play a simple song or whatever comes to mind. If possible, provide musical accompaniment either by singing along, playing along, or using recorded music. If this is too stressful for the person, play music and enjoy it with the person.

Dancing: Find recorded music from their past and have a dance – this activity helps strengthen muscles and preserve balance. Discuss the song; ask 'is that a trombone or a trumpet?' If this is too stressful for the person, give the person a scarf, tambourine, or shaker and allow the person to wave the object. Or have the person just watch everyone else dance and talk to the person about dance and what it means to him/her.

Watching a musical on video: This is a great activity; watch a movie from their past – the person can sing along or just enjoy watching the musical. If the person wishes, talk about the plot, make comments about the characters or actors, or talk about the scenery in the musical.

Listening to music (from their past): Popular music from one's past is often associated with happy events and can trigger important memories for a person. Many radio stations specialize in a specific era or genre.

Nature

Contact with nature provides benefits to persons with dementia including physical exercise, fresh air, and stimulation for all the senses.

Gardening: Planting a garden, weeding, raking leaves, and watering plants are all non-demanding activities an individual with dementia can do. It can be fun and productive for the person. Talk about what the plants are, when they will bloom, the type of fruits you will harvest, or if the person thinks the plants need watering. If the person is unable to perform gardening tasks, discuss gardening and talk about specific flowers or plants – if possible have pictures of plants/flowers.

Taking nature walks: Accompany the person on a walk and discuss the environment, scenic views, animals, and plants or leaves. Make sure to plan ahead and take along necessary items such as water and possibly food. Choose a route that does not exceed the person's abilities – avoid very long, strenuous walks. Consider taking a wheelchair in case the person tires. If this activity is too stressful, consider taking the person into the yard and talking about the trees, squirrels, or people driving by. If possible, make the route circular so the person ends back at the starting point; it is sometimes difficult to make a person with dementia turn around to return home.

Feeding fish, ducks, or birds: A simple pleasure can be feeding animals – fish, ducks, birds, or squirrels. Bring old bread and allow the person to toss small pieces to the animals. Allow the person to sit if possible to prevent tiring the person out. Talk about the animals, the weather, and your surroundings.

Collecting shells: If near a beach, collecting shells can allow a person to observe nature and get some exercise while picking up shells. Make sure the ocean does not frighten the person and that the person can physically walk on sand/uneven terrain. Talk about the shells and any memories from the person's past. If this is too stressful for the person, consider getting a bag of shells from a craft store; pour them on a table and ask the person which ones he/she would like to place in a bowl or would like to collect. Or sit near the beach and watch the ocean, the birds, and the people who are there.

Bird-watching: Bird-watching can be visually stimulating as well as allow the person to get outdoors. This can be done in a short walk, with the person in a wheelchair, or from a person's window. Place a birdfeeder where the person can bird-watch, a place to draw the birds for observation.

Watching fish in a fish tank or birds in a birdcage as well as outside the window: Watching beautiful, multicolored fish swim or birds fly around can be very relaxing and have a calming effect to reduce anxiety. Another option is to have books or pictures of animals to look at or discuss with the person. Even a trip to the pet store can be a stimulating activity for the person.

Helping Around the House

Individuals with dementia can develop feelings of uselessness and unproductiveness which can cause depression and diminish their quality of life. Keeping a person active and feeling as if they contribute to household chores will help prevent this problem and bring about satisfaction. Contributing to simple household chores can make a person with dementia feel more independent, feel better about him/herself, and improve their quality of life.

Helping with laundry: Do laundry at the same time every day or on the same days of the week to establish a routine. Allow the person to take laundry out of the dryer, separate and match socks, fold clothes from a basket, fold washcloths, or organize clothes. Talk about memories from their lives, such as who did the laundry or if they used a clothes line, etc.

Separating silverware or polishing silverware: This activity will exercise motor skills (remove knives and separate forks and spoons to make this task easier). Use a soft polish and monitor the person for putting it in their mouth. After the polish has dried, buff off the cream and remove tarnish. If this is too difficult, have the person separate silverware.

Sorting buttons: Sorting, cleaning, and organizing activities can help keep a person busy and bring back memories from his/her past. Ask a person to sort through a collection of buttons by shape, color, or size. Or sort nuts and bolts from a tool box, sort photos or children's toys. But monitor the person to make sure the objects are not put in their mouth. If this is too difficult, ask a person to tear strips of paper into 6-inch strips and put the strips in a bowl – demonstrate how to perform this task, and then allow the person to continue.

Washing the car: Ask the person to help wash, polish, or dry a car, if the person is physically capable of performing this task, but care should be taken to prevent spills, falls, or spraying; also, be safety conscious and monitor for fear of water Do not worry about the mess; clean up later. Or have the person come and keep the caregiver company while washing the car; talk to them during this activity.

Washing fruits & vegetables: Ask the person to separate fruits, potatoes or vegetables. Maybe ask the person to wash the fruit or vegetables in preparation for meals or snacks. Or allow the person to help by setting the table in preparation for meals.

If in a facility, some individuals with dementia can assist other residents to the dining area.

Stamping envelopes: Ask the person to help by placing stamps on envelops which need mailing. If this is too difficult, obtain rubber stamps, an ink pad, and some envelopes and allow the person to place the stamps on an envelope or a piece of paper.

Helping at mealtime: Activities the person may be able to perform include beating eggs, decorating a cake, filling sugar or creamer bowls, kneading bread, and setting the table. Remember step-by-step instructions and be cautious when around knives or other sharp objects, as well as mixers and stoves/ovens.

Making the bed: A daily routine can include making one's bed every day – this fosters a feeling of familiarity and comfort in repetition. Changing the sheets can be more challenging but can be a routine for the person. If this is too stressful, allow the person to help make the bed or just be there is observe and direct while the caregiver makes the bed.

Caring for houseplants: This can be a pleasurable and relaxing activity, as well as produce a feeling of productivity for a person. With help, the person can do many of the tasks related to plant care including repotting plants, watering or misting plants, and removing dead leaves or flowers.

Verbal Skills

Conversations can be frustrating for individuals with dementia. Normal exchanges with others can be loaded with information that the person can no longer remember or recall. Activities which stimulate verbal skills can help the person reconnect with other people.

Reading a story aloud: Reading newspapers, magazines, poems, or old letters is a good reading exercise. Individuals with dementia enjoy this type of routine as well as find it comforting. Make sure to keep distractions minimal, such as turning down the radio, television, or having the activity in a quiet area. Obtain large-print publications from libraries and the newspaper publishers. If the person is unable to read, read to the person and ask questions about what is being read.

Finding a country on a globe: Use a map or globe to stimulate conversations about islands, countries, or places. Discuss types of animals that reside there, weather conditions, what to wear there, or if the person has ever been there. If the person is unable to participate in such discussions, point out different places and talk to them about the places.

Dictating a letter: Ask the person to write a letter the caregiver dictates – either one you author or ask the person what they would like to say to a family member or friend and assist a person in writing that letter. If this is too difficult for the person or if the person is unable to write, have the person dictate a letter which the caregiver will write for him/her.

Talking about historic events: Since long-term memory is intact in many of the people with dementia, the person may find it enjoyable to discuss events from their past. Magazines such as American Heritage or National Geographic or old books which have information and pictures may spur discussions and memories. Old videos of important moments or periods of history are also good starting points for such conversations. Also remember, many old television series are now on DVD/CD and can tap into a person's memories.

<u>Asking for advice</u>: Older persons usually love to give advice. This activity engages the person and allows them to contribute. Ask their opinion or advice about a task, a person, a meal, or an activity. The question really does not matter; what matters is that you listen to the answer and let the person know you are listening by asking questions and/or repeating what you think the person said.

Games

Playing games can bring people together, reinforce social skills, and improve behavior. Individuals with dementia may not always remember the rules and may need to be prompted when it is their turn. Remember to be flexible with the rules if the person does not remember or becomes upset when corrected and reminded of the rules. The point of the game is the process of playing the game, engaging the person, and having fun.

<u>Bingo</u>: Use Bingo cards with large print and when the number is called, say the number verbally as well as have a large picture of the number so the person can see the number as well as hear it. Consider having some people play in teams or have someone assist the person in playing the game. Provide only simple prizes, such as a photograph or tissues.

<u>Crossword puzzles</u>: The caregiver may want to start a crossword puzzle (large print) and ask for help. Either have the person provide the answers or actually fill in the answers him/herself. If the person is unable to help provide the answers, discuss the questions and think through the answers by talking to the person about the answers.

<u>Jigsaw puzzles</u>: Some jigsaw puzzles have large pieces and bright colors – choose one with few pieces and simple designs. Ask the person to assemble the puzzle or hold a piece and ask the person where they think the piece should go.

Word games: Hidden words – find hidden words on a table – allow the person to assist in finding the words or play the game and point out to the person the words you find. Presidents – Match a president's first name with his last name.

Tossing a ball/beanbag: Find a comfortable place where the person can toss a ball or beanbag into a basket or through a large hole. Modify this activity by throwing the ball or beanbag back and forth to each other, or bounce the ball back and forth; or have the person squeeze a stress ball.

Treasure hunt: Fill a box with beans, corn, or rice and hide 'treasures' in the box – buttons, coins or any small objects. But be cautious the person does not place the objects in their mouth.

Draw a word: Match a word with a picture – either have the person do this or have the person direct and work together to match the word to the picture.

Card games: Play simple card games such as Go Fish or Old Maid – Use large print cards if possible. Sorting through sports cards is also good and can stimulate memories. Play a game where the person throwing down the highest card wins each hand – very simple rules are best but remember a person with dementia may not always play by the rules; be flexible and let them win.

Reminiscing

Remembering the past can be comforting and enjoyable for a person with dementia. Celebrating occasions is also a good way to trigger pleasurable memories as well as create new memories.

Celebrating a birthday: Birthday celebrations bring people together and can encourage reminiscing. The person can assist in preparing for the party or just be the one who is celebrated or wishes another person happy birthday.

<u>Taking a picture together</u>: Bring out funny hats, colorful outfits, or pets with which to have pictures taken. Take turns photographing each other and then enjoy the pictures together. Go somewhere and have pictures made. Talk about the pictures 'Remember this day when we had our picture made?'

<u>Celebrating a holiday</u>: Go beyond celebrating the big holidays and celebrate the smaller ones, as well as special days that you create - Arbor day, Columbus day, Mardi Gras (that's a fun one), May day, or Flag day. For Mardi Gras, have a parade and throw beaded necklaces and eat King Cake. For other holidays, plant a tree (or water a tree), read about Columbus, or make a May day basket.

<u>Putting a photo album together</u>: Bring out old photos, get pictures from magazines, and newspaper articles and ask the person to help organize them into a collection and/or album. Create a story about the photo and write it down near the picture, on a postcard or on the back of the picture for remembering later. Allow the person to organize the photos/pictures in the fashion they wish. Bring out this album later to allow the person to reminisce. If the person is unable to assist in this activity, have family or friends help put one together; include the stories to talk about with the person, and use this periodically to remind the person of their life.

<u>Stimulating a memory about the person's life (family or job)</u>: Create a designated 'office space' for the person to 'work'. They may be able to mimic their old jobs and feel productive again: for an accountant, provide a desk and calculator; for a beautician, provide combs, brushes, and curlers. Make sure to supervise the work activities, ask for productivity reports or schedules but when the person loses interest, remove the items/put them away and bring them out again at other times.

<u>Fashion</u>: Talk about the type of clothes the person once wore, ask about favorite outfits or colors, point out fashions in clothing catalogs, and have the person assist in choosing outfits he/she will wear (offer 2 to 3 choices to prevent overwhelming the person making a decision).

<u>Talking about childhood</u>: Reminiscing about childhood is often a very enjoyable activity for many elders. Ask about where he/she was born, where they grew up, where they went to school, and how many brothers/sisters they had. Ask about favorite childhood memories or something that made them laugh when they were a child. Be prepared for them to ask about relatives and friends who are no longer alive – do not stimulate grieving and discuss their deaths unless the person wants to talk about this subject and, if this topic seems to upset the person, allow them to discuss their feelings and/or distract the person's attention to another subject.

<u>Watching old movies or television shows</u>: Watching old movies or television shows can be fun and relaxing as it allows a person to connect with old memories, reminding the person of familiar stories, and is visually stimulating. Find old classic movies or television series on public television, on the internet or cable channels, or on DVD/CD. Choose movies or shows with which the person can connect. Discuss the actors, the plot, or anything which is in the show.

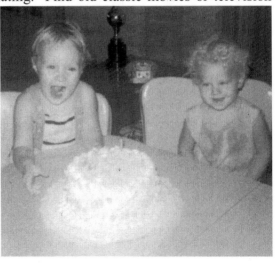

(Alzheimer's Activity Guide, 2005)

Hope

People suffering from dementia are facing serious illness and declines in their function. Families are experiencing a wide range of feelings as they watch their loved ones change. Death is a reality lurking around the corner. Through these harsh realities, hope has an important role. Hope isn't being unrealistic or denying problems. In some cases, hope can mean that things will improve tomorrow. In other cases, when improvement is unlikely, hope offers the assurance that one will be able to face whatever occurs tomorrow: comfort will be offered, support will be provided, and one will not be alone. The encouraging words and hope can help you face another day. AALTCN, (2010)

Chapter 12 References

AALTCN. (2010). Affirmations. Retrieved March 23, 2010 from emails American Association of Long Term care Nurses Newsletter.

AllLaw.com. (2010). Living Will. Retrieved March 22, 2010 from http://www.alllaw.com/articles/wills_and_trusts/article7.asp

Alzheimer's Activities Guide: In It Together. (2005). A publication of Forrest Pharmaceuticals, Inc.

Boyles, F. (2006). *Coach Broyles Playbook for Alzheimer's Caregivers: A Practical Tips Guide*. Fayetteville, Arkansas.

Burggraf, V., Duffy, E., & Engel, S. (2008). Alzheimer's Disease: Caring for the Caregiver. *Counseling Points*. 1(3).

Caregiver Guide. (2010). Retrieved March 23, 2010 from http://www.nia.nih.gov/Alzheimers/Publications/caregiverguide.htm#intro

Courtney, R. (2008). *Essential planning guide for families dealing with dementia*. Jackson, Mississippi.

Family Caregiver Alliance (2010). Communication tips. Retrieved April 9, 2010 from http://www.nia.nih.gov/nia.nih.gov/Templates/ADEARCommon/ADEARCommonPage.aspx?NRMODE=Published&NRNODEGUID=%7bC2F11D41-E5FE-435D-9C9D-A3489319D4AD%7d&NRORIGINALURL=%2fAlzheimers%2fPublications%2fcaregiverguide%2ehtm&NRCACHEHINT=Guest#communication

Fisher Center for Alzheimer's Research. (2010). Alzheimer's Therapeutic Activities. Retrieved April 11, 2010 from http://www.alzinfo.org/alzheimers-treatment-therapeutic.asp

Fraser, M. (2007). Caring for Caregivers. *ElderCare*. 7(2):10-12.

Help Guide (2010). End of Life Care. Retrieved April 29, 2010 from http://helpguide.org/elder/alzheimers_disease_dementia_caring_final_stage.htm

Keane, B. (2003). Montessori principles work for Alzheimer's: what did Maria Montessori discover in her work with children that could be useful in the care of residents with Alzheimer's or other dementias? Nursing Homes. Retrieved April 11, 2010 from http://findarticles.com/p/articles/mi_m3830/is_6_52/ai_103194330/

Sellman, J. (2010). Hospice Care and Alzheimer's disease. About. com Retrieved May 3, 2010 from http://alzheimers.about. com/lw/Health-Medicine/Conditions-and-diseases/Hospice-Care-and-Alzheimers.htm

Chapter 13

Late Stage or Terminal Dementia

In the final stages of a dementia (including Alzheimer's disease), there is a shift of care priorities and focus is on comfort care. Caregivers may experience grieving over the loss of the person even before their physical death. The complex and often disorderly progression of this terminal disease can make the journey to the person's final days difficult as the person reaches the stage where he/she requires complete care 24 hours a day, 7 days a week. Simple acts of daily care, such as bathing, feeding, turning, and cleaning the person; contrast with complex end-of-life decisions, such as whether to institute or continue life-prolonging medical care; and profound bereavement. Caregivers can learn to anticipate, remember, and reconnect with the person, which may ease the journey through care and grief.

Introduction

In the final or terminal stages of a person's dementia, it becomes evident that in spite of the best care, attention, and treatment, the person is approaching the end of life. At this stage, the individual can no longer communicate directly, is totally dependent on others for all activities of daily living, such as turning, grooming, and eating, and is generally confined to bed. The person is unable to recognize people (family, friends, and caregivers) or to verbally express their wants, needs, and problems. Many caregivers may finally be forced to acknowledge their own needs for significant help. Understanding and anticipating the physical and psychological changes which likely will occur will help caregivers in offering quality care in the person's final days

Physical Changes in Terminal Stage of Dementia

The person:
- Forgets who the caregiver is
- Forgets who the person is
- Is unable to make sense when talking
- Is unable to walk
- Is unable to sit up
- Is unable to control bowel or bladder
- Is unable to understand what the person is seeing
  The person may be limited to grunts & groans; the muscles in the person's face do not work anymore, the person may cry or laugh inappropriately, they will be unable to turn over in bed; they may lean to one side when sitting up, they may fall over in chair if not propped up; or they may be limited to chair or bed.

What you can do for the person at in the terminal stage of dementia
- Love the person
- Touch often
- Reassure often
- Change body position every 2 hours
- Gently rub person's skin if areas are reddened
- Use a Geri-Chair which can be put in several positions
- Make sure clothing is not bunched up
- Use pillows or a wedge to prop person upright

Although cognitive and memory functions are greatly diminished, a person in the final stages of dementia may still have the capacity to feel frightened or at peace, loved or lonely, and sad or secure. It is believed that hearing is the last sensory function to be lost. The most helpful interventions are those which aim to promote comfort and provide human contact as well as meaningful connections to others. The following are the physical changes which occur and some suggestions for addressing these issues.

Physical Changes in Terminal Dementia

System	Changes	Helpful Hints
Muscles	• Muscles stop working • Muscles begin to waste & atrophy • Curl up in fetal position (like a baby) • Joints become stiff • Forget how to sit up	• Be gentle when moving the person • Slowly unbend arms & legs • Give medicine for pain • If the person can help hold weight, stand them up • Assist with pivoting to chair
Skin	• Loses elasticity – does not stretch as readily • Bruises easily • Skin tears easily occur • Pressure areas easily develop on boney prominences such as elbows, hips, heels, & bottom as well as between knees	• Gently touch & move the person when changing positions • Keep skin clean • Keep arms, legs, elbows, & back moist with lotion • Use soft booties to keep heels off the bed • Change the person's position every 2 hours • Check skin frequently (tears, redness, sores) Gently rub & lotion red areas • Mark red spots & note size • Assess red areas for softness or bogginess (see if skin area feels mushy) • Keep weight off red spots • Use special mattress cover designed to protect skin

System	Changes	Helpful Hints
Bowel & Bladder changes	• Lose bowel & bladder control • Unable to completely empty bladder • Forget what sensations mean (to void or have bowel movement)	• Check the person at least every 2 hours to keep the person's skin clean • Monitor bowel movements- the person should have at least 3 bowel movements per week (if no bowel movement, a laxative or suppository may be used to stimulate the person's bowels to move)
Mouth	• Tongue dry • Mouth tastes bad • Unable to ask for water or clean own teeth • Cannot follow directions to rinse & spit • Cannot open mouth when asked • Dentures do not fit due to weight loss	• Never force the person's mouth open • Take dentures out if they do not fit • Use soft toothbrush to clean teeth, gums, & tongue • Use very little toothpaste or fluid to prevent choking when performing mouth care • Put on side so fluid can run out of mouth • Use small amounts of glycerin on tongue to increase spit in mouth • Offer small sips of water throughout the day • Put petroleum jelly on lips

End of Life Decisions

The terminal stage of dementia often presents many issues which must be addressed and are often more difficult for family members than individuals, since the person with dementia is no longer aware of his/her surroundings. Sometimes intricate and highly personal decisions can be difficult and emotional. Sometimes the focus is shifted from issues about comfort and dignity to issues about guilt and unresolved personal or relationship issues of family members.

Focus on values. If a person in the final stages or terminal stage of dementia did not prepare a living will or advanced directives while competent to do so, caregivers are encouraged to act on what the person would have wished. To the extent possible, consider treatment, placement, and decisions about dying from the person's preferences and from the person's point of view.

Family conflicts: Family members vary in their understanding of the dementing disease processes and the capacities of a person suffering from dementia for emotional openness and expression. When stress and grief are heightened by the person's deterioration and withdrawal, conflict can result amongst family members. If families are unable to agree on living arrangements, medical treatment, or end-of-life directives, ask a trained healthcare professional, social worker, or hospice specialist for mediation assistance. Prolonged disagreement can impact the caregiver's ability to grieve and hamper well-being.

Communicate: Choosing one person who will be the primary decision maker and communicator to manage information facilitates family involvement and support. Even when families know the person's wishes, implementing decisions for or against sustaining or life-prolonging treatments requires communication and coordination.

If children are involved, assess their ability to understand and gauge their emotional needs, but make efforts to include them as much as possible. Children manage these situations better if families offer

325

honest, developmentally appropriate information about the person's condition and the children are prepared for the approaching death. Children can be deeply affected by situations they don't understand, and may benefit by expressing their feelings and emotions through drawing pictures or keeping a journal, and hearing stories that explain the situation and events in terms they can grasp (HelpGuide, 2010).

Hospice

As of 2010, Alzheimer's disease became the sixth leading cause of death in the United States, and the number of families caring for someone with this progressive brain disorder is only expected to grow as the population ages (Sellman, 2010). When a person is within the last 6 month to a year of life, some individuals in terminal dementia are referred to Hospice. This is a service which assists the person as well as the family through the final days. Their focus is on quality of life, helping with comfort measures, and dignity while going through a dying process. The shift in care begins with accepting the upcoming event, death. The first step is letting go of the person – accept that the person's death is approaching and work towards comfort management. **To be eligible for hospice care, a person with a diagnosis of Alzheimer's disease must also be:**

- unable to walk unassisted
- unable to dress him/herself
- unable to bathe or perform grooming needs without help
- unable to control bowel and bladder
- unable to converse effectively (though some language may remain)

In addition, the individual must have recently had at least one serious health issue, such as a severe respiratory or kidney infection, evidence of profound nutritional problems, or severe open bedsores (Sellman, 2010).

Questions about Comfort Care in a Terminally Ill Individual Suffering from Alzheimer's Disease

---

Is the person experiencing hunger or thirst?
- Most researchers believe that a person in the final stage of dementia does not sense or understand the sensations of hunger or thirst
- Feeding tubes will not prevent weight loss nor significantly improve the nutritional status of a person in the terminal stage of dementia

Is the person experiencing pain?
- Some individuals in the terminal stage of dementia still experience pain and discomfort until they are no longer aware of their surroundings or their own body's needs
- Subtle behavioral changes can signal unmet needs such as pain, constipation, or other discomforts: The person may grimace, grunt, grab, or moan
- Managing pain and discomfort requires daily monitoring and reassessment of subtle nonverbal signals
- Be alert for a significant decline in a person's functioning
  » Some families choose to discontinue other medical interventions

Depression
- Symptoms may include sadness or crying as well as refusing to eat or cooperate in care
- Manage depression by spending time with the person and talking to the person or singing; touch is also very important
- Depression and/or anxiety may need to be managed with medication to improve quality of life for the person

Sleep problems
- The person may sleeping all day or staying awake all night
- As much as possible, interact with the person during daytime hours, and have a set bedtime routine so the person sleeps better

327

Eventually, the person in the final stage of dementia will die. The cause of death will be Alzheimer's disease, but the direct cause may be due to dehydration, heart failure, or infection – most commonly a urinary tract infection or a respiratory infection. Usually, the person becomes dehydrated because he/she is not alert enough to eat or drink.

Signs and Symptoms of Dehydration
- Poor skin turgor
- Sunken eyes
- Decreased level of consciousness
- Increased confusion, combativeness, or aggression
- Increase risk for Urinary tract infections

Grieving may continue after physical death occurs. Some caregivers experience a devastating loss even though they were aware that death was imminent. And some caregivers experience a sense of relief because they know the person is no longer suffering and is in a better place. But every caregiver will have physical and emotional needs while in the midst of caring for a dying individual and experiencing the loss of the person. Support groups can provide help through the grieving process. And every caregiver needs to remember, there is no such thing as a perfect caregiver, they did the best they could do and were there when the person needed them the most.

Caring for the Caregiver

As impossible as it may seem, taking care of the caregiver during a person's final stages of life is critically important. Research shows spousal caregivers are more likely to experience despair while adult children find fulfillment through their caregiving roles (Help Guide, 2010). Acceptance and allowing oneself to grieve is important to be able to adjust, feel whole again, and move on.

From the moment of a diagnosis of dementia, a caregiver's life is never the same. The journey does not end in the person's death; caregivers must work through a grieving process before it is truly completed. Replacing lost relationships, using these experiences to help others, and gaining new perspective will help return to some caregivers to a sense of normalcy.

Reconnect

- Join a bereavement support group. Be with others who are going through or have gone through the death of a family member, can understand emotions and offer support through these difficult times
- Enroll in an adult education class such as yoga, Tai-Chi, exercise classes, or art classes. Acquiring new skills and staying physically active will promote healing.
- Try a new group, such as a book club, volunteer, or start a neighborhood bunco group. Learn to enjoy, laugh, and connect; such emotional and social needs continue after the person is gone.
- Talk to a therapist or grief counselor if necessary. The key is to give oneself permission to find new meaning and relationships; this can be difficult, but acceptance and moving forward are steps to health and happiness.

Acts of love and connections can sustain the person who had a battle with dementia through a long and difficult passage. To assist in the healing after the loss of the person, caregivers should be encouraged to share what was learned, cultivate happiness, and find new meaning in order to build a loving finale to the caregiving journey.

Chapter 13 References

Affirmations – AALTCN. (2010) Retrieved March 23, 2010 from emails American Association of Long Term care Nurses Newsletter.

Caregiver Guide. (2010). Retrieved March 23, 2010 from http://www.nia.nih.gov/Alzheimers/Publications/caregiverguide.htm#intro

Courtney, R. (2008). *Essential planning guide for families dealing with dementia.* Jackson, Mississippi.

Help Guide (2010). End of Life Care. Retrieved April 29, 2010 from http://helpguide.org/elder/alzheimers_disease_dementia_caring_final_stage.htm

Sellman, J. (2010). Hospice Care and Alzheimer's disease. About. com Retrieved May 3, 2010 from http://alzheimers.about.com/lw/Health-Medicine/Conditions-and-diseases/Hospice-Care-and-Alzheimers.htm

Chapter 14

The End of Mom's Story

A conclusion to our long journey will be shared and lessons learned from the experience.

The Ending to Mom's Story

Mom had been diagnosed with colon cancer many years before. She agreed to 6 months of chemotherapy but would do no more. We would take her there, hold her hand until they started her IV for the chemotherapy and help her through this very difficult time. The chemotherapy and the medications she had to take to manage the symptoms related to chemo made her feel horrible – increasing her confusion, making her experience more pain and anorexia, and it didn't really help. At the end of 6 months, the CT scan showed a new spot on her lung. She made the choice not to continue with chemo treatments and let whatever was going to happen, happen. We went on doing relatively okay for another 7 years (pretty good considering she had a large mass – the size of a grapefruit and it had already metastasized to lymph nodes).

She lived a fairly normal life and was independent as long as possible, but one summer, she told me about the growing lump in her breast. She did not wish to have any medical evaluation or treatment since she 'would not go through chemo again.' The lump was fairly large when she allowed me to look; it had already spread to both breasts – the progression was very rapid. We finally went to a surgeon when the pain became unbearable – the diagnosis was inflammatory breast cancer. She was placed on Hospice at home to help us manage her pain.

We had also noticed she was off-balance a bit and she began to fall occasionally. When the falling became more frequent, we took turns staying with her to help prevent falls or help her up if she did fall. She would have her days and night mixed up, staying awake all night and sleeping all day. My wonderful niece, who had begun nursing school, agreed to move in with her to have someone around (she was wonderful to my Mom – her grandmother – and we really couldn't have made it through this without her!) Mom was able to stay at home and maintained this way of life for almost 6 more months. Then things got really bad.

Mom was confused and scared. She would forget things frequently and had frequent mood swings. We made every attempt to keep her home, but when she stayed awake for almost 3 weeks straight – napping only short periods of time, she wore all three of us out (my sister, my niece, and me). One of us would be sitting on the couch, nodding off and would hear a thud in the bedroom from where Mom had crawled out of bed, over the bedrail of the hospital bed we had moved to her house. We made the decision to move her to an inpatient Hospice Center. This was one of the hardest things we have ever had to do. We had talked about the possibility of placing her in a nursing home, but she adamantly did not want to go to any place like that. So, it took a lot for us to do this, but I am very glad we did. She received the care she needed and the companionship she desired. I began cleaning out her house between visits to Hospice, working, and family – it allowed me to experience her life and work towards bringing things to closure. I did a lot of grieving at this time, long before the physical death ensued.

The staff at the Hospice center was very special and they worked to make Mom feel special too, even though she was confused, would stay up all night with the nightshift nurses and help them 'chart' – she was right at home thinking she was back at work in a hospital – she felt needed.
At first Mom was not happy to be there, but she was where she needed to be – she was wearing everyone out – herself

included. We thought there was a possibility we could get her days and nights straightened out, get her pain under control, and get her back home. But this was not in our future. She continued to decline, physically as well as cognitvely. Sometimes Mom knew me, sometimes I was a familiar nurse co-worker or a friend, and sometimes she really did not know me at all. I would visit routinely to bring her favorite foods (sweets – especially anything chocolate; strawberries and Cokes were her favorites). I would help her eat, feed her, or just watch television with her and tell her about my day.

She lost weight and became more and more confused, trying to get out of bed and falling frequently at the Hospice center too. At first, Mom could walk with assistance, but this rapidly declined. Some days she would not eat or drink anything at all – she could go for 2 weeks without eating and only taking sips of water. Then, she would miraculously come back to herself, talking as if nothing had happened – back to her baseline confusion. This went on for months. But the episodes of not eating and drinking became more and more frequent. She had gone from a size 20 to a size 8 – we were buying her several new gowns and comfortable clothes to wear. Approaching the final months, I would just go sit and read the paper to her – sometimes she acted like she was paying attention and other times she did not.

The final week came; I had a planned work trip, which was out of town. She had not been very alert that week, but I was only to be out of town for a couple of days; she had done this many times before and come back out of it. But this time, something told me this might be the last time I would see her alive, so I said a goodbye even though I wasn't sure she heard me. The following day, I received a call that she was not doing well and she was near her final hours. My sister and niece rushed to the Hospice. Mom went quietly and peacefully.

Epilogue

I tried to get back quickly, but there wasn't much I could really do. My sister helped make the arrangements for the service (Mom had already decided what she wanted and we knew what steps to take to follow her wishes). Now Mom was giving until the end, she donated her body to science, so we had a funeral mass and celebration of her life. I did cry a little but I almost feel guilty for not 'breaking down' and sobbing uncontrollably. I think I did most of my grieving before she actually died and the physical death was almost a relief – she was no longer suffering and I know she now had her faculties back.

Mom – I miss her greatly. Not a day goes by that I do not think about her. My journey is not over yet; I am still working through a few things, but I am on the final road. This book was a part of my journey. This was my attempt to help others through education, examples which bring the disease to life, experiences based on my professional and personal life, and sharing my story of Mom to offer support to others who might be going through what I spent 10 years going through and being a caregiver with this wonderful person.

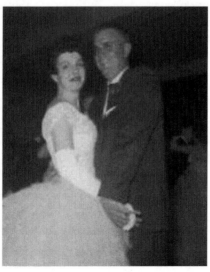

Lessons learned:

1. No control: Caregivers cannot stop a progressive disease; the disease will continue to advance. Sometimes, even with best efforts, a caregiver cannot control the person or their behaviors.
2. Flexibility: A person will not behave the way a caregiver expects or will not respond the way a caregiver expects, even varying their responses to a technique that worked the last time.
3. Patience: A person's disease and dementia will advance at a pace the caregiver cannot control. Patience is a virtue that will help in going through these processes.
4. Life is precious: Life can be quantified by length of life as well as quality of life. A person's life must be lived the way the person wishes it to be lived – caregivers must respect an individual for their choices in the direction of their own life.

Thank you for reading and GOOD LUCK!

Now that this part of my journey has come to an end, I think I can finally cry now.

Appendix A

Medications commonly used to treat problematic behaviors associated with dementia

Medication	Geriatric Dosage Suggestions	Potential Side Effects of Medication
Cholinesterase Inhibitors *indicated for treatment of the early, middle, & late stages of Alzheimer's disease; Rivastigmine is also indicated by the FDA to treat Parkinson's disease dementia*		
donepezil (Aricept)	5 mg daily for 30 days then 10 mg daily *23mg daily dose available in certain individuals after the person has been on Aricept 10mg daily for a minimum of 3 months	Most common problems are related to loss of appetite, nausea, vomiting, abdominal pain, and diarrhea
rivastigmine (Exelon)	start @ 1.5 twice a day for 2 weeks, then 3 mg twice a day for 2 weeks, then 4.5 mg twice a day, then 6 mg twice a day (max dose - 12 mg/day); *Patch is available = 4.6 mg/24 hour – change once a day for 1 month, then increase to 9.5 mg/24 hour	
galantamine (Razadyne)	4 mg twice a day, increase every 4 weeks until reaching12 mg twice a day	
N–Methyl D – Aspartate Receptor Antagonists *indicated by the FDA for treating the middle and late stages of Alzheimer's disease*		
memantine (Namenda)	Titration: Start at 5 mg daily for 7 days, then 5 mg twice a day for 7 days, then 5 mg in morning, 10 mg in evening for 7 days, then 10 mg twice a day	Sedation, constipation, dizziness, headache, and pain

Continued on page 338

Appendix A

Antidepressants – Selective Seratonin Reuptake Inhibitors (SSRI)		
indicated by the FDA to treat depression		
bupropion (Wellbutrin)	75-100 mg once a day or twice a day	**Entire Class of SSRI: Weight gain, dizziness, somnolence, insomnia, decreased libido, tremors, akathesia, nervousness, sweating, and various gastrointestinal, as well as sexual, disturbances
citalopram (Celexa)	20-40 mg once a day	
duloxetine (Cymbalta)	20-60 mg once a day	
escitalopram (Lexapro)	5-20 mg once a day	
fluoxetine (Prozac)	10-20 mg once a day	
paroxetine (Paxil)	10-40 mg once a day	
paroxetine CR (Paxil CR)	12.5-37.5 mg once a day	
sertraline (Zoloft)	25-50 mg once a day	
venlafaxine XR (Effexor XR)	37.5-150 mg once a day	
Anxiolytics *indicated by the FDA for treatment of anxiety symptoms –* **Not recommended to routinely use anxiolytics**		
alprazolam (Xanax)	0.25-0.5 mg every 6 to 8 hours as needed	Sedation, falls, orthostatic hypotension & increased confusion
clonazepam (Klonipin)	0.125-2 mg every 12 hours as needed (*has a long half-life)	
clorazepapte (Tranxene)	3.75-15 mg every 8 hours as needed	
lorazepam (Ativan)	0.5-2mg every 6 to 8 hours as needed (*has the shortest half-life and is the drug of choice if necessary in elders with dementia if ultimately necessary)	

Antipsychotic medications *not indicated by the FDA for treating behavioral problems in elders with dementia; Indicated for use with agitation and psychosis in individuals with psychosis, bipolar disorder and other psychiatric conditions*		
aripiprazole (Abilify)	2-30 mg once or twice a day	Hypotension, seizures, hyperglycemia, worsening of diabetes, weight gain, headache, cataract formation, worsening of depression, & hyperprolactinemia
olanzapine (Zyprexa)	1.25-10 mg once a day at bedtime or twice a day	
quetiapine (Seroquel)	12.5-200 mg once, twice or three times a day	
risperidone (Risperdal)	0.25 to 1 mg once or twice a day	*Antipsychotic medications have the potential to cause sedation, somnolence or insomnia, orthostatic hypotension, falls, strokes, diabetes, extrapyramidal symptoms, dystonic movements, myocardial infarction, and death
ziprasidone (Geodon)	20-80 mg once or twice a day QT prolongation, hypertension, rash * must monitor EKGs	
		**all patients receiving drugs in this class must have routine monitoring of liver & kidney functioning, Hgb A1C, Cholesterol
all patients receiving drugs in this class must have routine monitoring of liver & kidney functioning, Hgb A1C, Cholesterol		

Continued on page 340

Appendix A

Seizure medication (used for its side effect of calming behavioral problems) *indicated by the FDA for treatment of seizure disorder and not indicated by the FDA for use of managing behavioral problems in elders with dementia*		
divalproic acid (Depakote)	125-500 mg once or twice a day	Somnolence, dizziness, falls, orthostatic hypotension, increased confusion, & liver toxicity *all patients receiving this medication must have routine monitoring of Liver functioning and Depakote levels

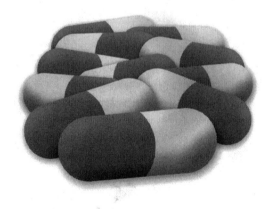

Appendix B

Neuropsychiatric Testing

Neuropsychiatric testing involves having a person with questionable cognitive functioning answer questions and perform tasks that have been carefully designed for the purpose of assessing cognition and the presence of a psychiatric and/or neurological disorder. It is carried out by a specialist who has been educated and trained in administering this examination. Neuropsychological testing addresses an individual's appearance, mood, anxiety level, and experience of delusions or hallucinations. Neuropsychological testing gives a more accurate diagnosis of these types of problems and thus can help in treatment planning. The tests are repeated periodically to see how well treatments are working as well as to check for new problems (eMedicine, 2010).

Information Obtained from Neuropsychological Reports

Neuropsychological tests are a series of measures that identify cognitive impairment and functioning in individuals. They provide quantifiable data about the following aspects of cognition:

- Reasoning and problem solving ability
- Ability to understand and express language
- Working memory and attention
- Short-term and long-term memory
- Processing speed
- Visual-spatial organization
- Visual-motor coordination
- Planning, synthesizing, and organizing abilities

Established Applications of Neuropsychological Evaluation (NPE)

Applications of NPE include the following:

- Provide a differential diagnosis of organic and functional pathologies
- Assess for dementia versus pseudodementia
- Determine the presence of epilepsy versus somatoform disorder
- Determine the presence of traumatic brain injury sequelae versus malingering or unconscious highlighting
- Guide rehabilitation programs and monitor patient progress
- Guide the therapist in referring to specialists
- Provide data to guide decisions about the patient's condition, such as the following:
  - Competency to manage legal and financial affairs
  - Capacity to participate in medical and legal decision-making
  - Ability to live independently or with supervision
  - Ability to return to work and school affairs
  - Candidacy for transplants
- Provide data to guide the following assessments and procedures:
  - Evaluation of the cognitive effects of various medical disorders and associated interventions
  - Assessment of tests for diabetes mellitus, chronic obstructive pulmonary disease (COPD), hypertension, human immunodeficiency virus (HIV) infection, coronary artery bypass graft (CABG), and clinical drug trials
  - Assessment of CNS lesions and/or seizure disorders before and after surgical interventions, including corpus callosotomy, focal resection (e.g., topectomy, lobectomy), and multiple subpial transection
  - Monitoring the effects of pharmacologic interventions

o Documenting the cognitive effects of exposure to neurotoxins

o Documenting adverse effects of whole brain irradiation in children

o Comparing with guidelines for electroconvulsive therapy (ECT) influenced by standardized evaluation of memory

o Standard protocols for assessment of specific disorders, such as dementia of the Alzheimer type (DAT), multiple sclerosis (MS), TBI, and stroke

o Developmental disorders (e.g., specific learning disabilities) require detailed assessment of cognition, academic achievement, and psychosocial adjustment for proper identification and as a guide to their management. Academic placement in special education and resource classrooms may be needed.

NPE is of limited value in the following cases:

- The individual is severely compromised, as in advanced dementia or early in recovery from serious brain injury, although brief serial assessment with measures such as the Galveston Orientation and Amnesia Test, high-velocity lead therapy, digit span, and motor speed and dexterity is very useful in tracking recovery.
- The individual has other serious medical complications or psychiatric disorders.

Appendix B Reference

Malik, A., Turner, M., & Sadler, C. (2010). Neuropsychologial Evaluation. eMedicine.net, Retrieved May 3, 2010 from http://emedicine.medscape.com/article/317596-overview

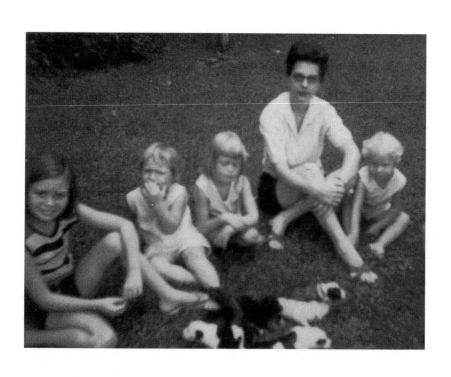

Definitions & Terms

Ageism: is a type of stereotyping – a belief about elders which views aging individuals as having an expectation to become senile, confused, demented.

Alzheimer's disease: A pathological disorder of the brain which causes chemical changes in a person's brain, cognitive impairment, and eventual shrinkage of the brain. The person develops strange clumps of protein (plaques) and tangled fibers inside the nerve cells of his brain.

Anomia: difficulty naming objects.

Anosmia: a diminished sense of smell.

Anxious Symptoms: Anxiety; Restlessness; Chronic complaints – i.e., pain, constipation, insomnia, etc.; Muscle irritability; Irritability; Concentration problems; Headaches, backaches or digestive problems; Insomnia.

Aphasia: difficulty using and/or understanding language.

Auditory hallucination: hearing sounds or people talking which are not real; Some people who experience auditory hallucinations that occur where the individual has conversations with people (who are not really there) including deceased loved ones.

Delirium: a sudden severe confusion and rapid changes in mentation of a person – occurring over a few hours to a few days with markedly increased changes in level of consciousness, including confusion and agitation.

Delusion: a belief about an event that is untrue, but the event is not out of context with a person's social and cultural background.

Delusional misidentification: may result from a combined decline in visual function and recent memory problems – individuals may suspect that a family member is an impostor, believe that strangers are living in their home, or fail to recognize their own reflection in a mirror.

Dementia: not a disease itself, but a group of symptoms caused by various diseases or conditions with symptoms which include changes in personality, mood, and behavior. It is the loss of mental functions such as thinking, memory, and reasoning which is severe enough to interfere with a person's ability to carry out the daily tasks of living.

Depressed Symptoms: No interest or pleasure in things the person used to enjoy; Feeling sad or numb; Crying easily or for no reason; Feeling slowed down; Feeling worthless or guilty; Change in appetite; unintended change in weight; Trouble recalling things, concentrating or making decisions; Problems sleeping, or wanting to sleep all of the time; Feeling tired all of the time; Thoughts about death or suicide.

Disinhibition: a lack of social skills and restraint to adhere to social norms, which manifest in several ways, including disregard for acceptable behaviors, poor risk assessment, and impulsivity; an individual suffering from dementia is less able to exercise normal control – to choose to inhibit some responses in the way most people would do each day for reasons of politeness, sensitivity, social appropriateness, or desire to keep our true feelings hidden from others.

Durable Power of Attorney: a document which assigns another individual to make medical decisions and authorizes that person to make financial decisions. This allows another person to make decisions regarding healthcare and to sign medical consent forms. This also allows the individual access to the person's bank accounts and finances, gives authority to sell property, and make decisions regarding the person's living environment. A person authorizes this while he/she is legally capable of making decisions and the document is filed in a Court of Law in the county/state where the person resides.

Durable Financial Power of Attorney: a document which authorizes another individual to make only financial decisions. This allows another individual access to bank accounts and finances and gives that individual authority to sell property. The person suffering from dementia authorizes this while he/she is legally capable of making decisions and the document filed in a Court of Law in the county/state where the person resides.

Dyarthria: a problem where physically producing speech is difficult.

Dystonia: a neurological movement disorder, in which sustained muscle contractions cause twisting and repetitive movements or abnormal postures.

Guardianship: a legal manner in which a person who is unable to make decisions has another individual make decisions for him/her. If a person is no longer competent to make decisions due to Alzheimer's disease or another disease process – if there is no Advanced Directive or Durable Power of Attorney in place, and if there is not a relative who is available to make decisions for the individual – the courts will assign a Guardian to make medical and financial decisions for the person.

Hallucination: a false sensory perception that is not merely distortions or misinterpretations; Auditory hallucinations are hearing sounds or voices which are not real; Visual hallucinations are seeing objects, colors, or visions which are not real.

Hyperphagia: disinhibition with social conventions to repress placing objects in a person's mouth. Can be expressed as behaviors such as constantly eating, placing things in mouth, chewing constantly, or smacking lips frequently.

Hypersexuality: disinhibition with social conventions to repress sexual urges. Can be expressed with behaviors such as being preoccupied sexual demand or with fondling self or others.

Mild Cognitive Impairment (MCI): a level of cognitive or memory impairment beyond that which usually occurs in individuals normally as they age, but not truly a type of "dementia" or "Alzheimer's disease".

Nonpharmacologic interventions: the foundation of care, including creating a simplistic and safe environment, a predictable routine, counseling for caregivers about the unintentional nature of psychotic symptoms, and offering strategies to manage as well as cope with troubling behaviors.

Prosopagnosia: difficulty recognizing faces.

Sad or Depressed Symptoms: No interest or pleasure in things you used to enjoy; Feeling sad or numb; Crying easily or for no reason; Feeling slowed down; Feeling worthless or guilty; Change in appetite; unintended change in weight; Trouble recalling things, concentrating or making decisions; Problems sleeping, or wanting to sleep all of the time; Feeling tired all of the time; Thoughts about death or suicide.

Self-neglect: Individuals who do not eat right, do not pay attention to personal hygiene, or have issues sleeping – too much or too little, or exhibit behavioral problems.

'Senility': also referred to as dementia – the loss of mental functions such as thinking, memory, and reasoning which is severe enough to interfere with a person's ability to carry out the daily tasks of living.

Sundowning behaviors: behavioral problems a person with a diagnosis of dementia can express caused by a physiological disease/dementia and can include aggression, agitation, apathy, repetitive behaviors, suspicion, and wandering.

Visual hallucinations: can range from seeing abstract shapes or colors to visions of animals and people which are not really present.

Other troubling issues: can include **non-psychotic behaviors** associated with dementia: agitation, wandering, sexual disinhibition, and aggression.

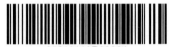
35210119R00204

Made in the USA
San Bernardino, CA
17 June 2016